SpringerBriefs in Statistics

SpringerBriefs in Statistics - ABE

SpringerBriefs present concise summaries of cutting-edge research and practical applications across a wide spectrum of fields. Featuring compact volumes of 50 to 125 pages, the series covers a range of content from professional to academic. Briefs are characterized by fast, global electronic dissemination, standard publishing contracts, standardized manuscript preparation and formatting guidelines, and expedited production schedules.

Typical topics might include:

- A timely report of state-of-art techniques
- A bridge between new research results, as published in journal articles, and a contextual literature review
- A snapshot of a hot or emerging topic
- An in-depth case study
- A presentation of core concepts that students must understand in order to make independent contributions

This SpringerBriefs in Statistics – ABE subseries aims to publish relevant contributions to several fields in the Statistical Sciences, produced by full members of the ABE – Associação Brasileira de Estatística (Brazilian Statistical Association), or by distinguished researchers from all Latin America. These texts are targeted to a broad audience that includes researchers, graduate students and professionals, and may cover a multitude of areas like Pure and Applied Statistics, Actuarial Science, Econometrics, Quality Assurance and Control, Computational Statistics, Risk and Probability, Educational Statistics, Data Mining, Big Data and Confidence and Survival Analysis, to name a few.

More information about this subseries at http://www.springer.com/subseries/13778

Víctor Hugo Lachos Dávila
Celso Rômulo Barbosa Cabral
Camila Borelli Zeller

Finite Mixture of Skewed Distributions

ABE

Springer

Víctor Hugo Lachos Dávila
Department of Statistics
University of Connecticut
Storrs Mansfield, CT, USA

Celso Rômulo Barbosa Cabral
Department of Statistics
Federal University of Amazonas
Manaus, Brazil

Camila Borelli Zeller
Department of Statistics
Federal University of Juiz de Fora
Juiz de Fora, Minas Gerais, Brazil

ISSN 2191-544X ISSN 2191-5458 (electronic)
SpringerBriefs in Statistics
ISSN 2524-6917
SpringerBriefs in Statistics – ABE
ISBN 978-3-319-98028-7 ISBN 978-3-319-98029-4 (eBook)
https://doi.org/10.1007/978-3-319-98029-4

Library of Congress Control Number: 2018951927

Mathematics Subject Classification: 62-07, 62Exx, 62Fxx, 62Jxx

This Springer imprint is published by the registered company Springer Nature Switzerland AG
The registered company address is: Gewerbestrasse 11, 6330 Cham, Switzerland

Lourdes, Carlos e Marcelo (Camila Borelli Zeller)
Sílvia, Ivanete e Gabriela (Celso Rômulo Barbosa Cabral)
Rosa Dávila, Eduardo, Thuany e Alberto (Víctor Hugo Lachos Dávila)

Preface

Modeling based on finite mixture distributions is a rapidly developing area with an exploding range of applications. Finite mixture models are nowadays applied in such diverse areas as biology, biometrics, genetics, medicine, and marketing, among others. The main objective of this book is to present recent results in this area of research, which intended to prepare the readers to undertake mixture models using scale mixtures of skew-normal (SMSN) distributions. We consider maximum likelihood estimation for univariate and multivariate finite mixtures where components are members of the flexible class of SMSN distributions proposed by Lachos et al. (2010), which is a subclass of the skew-elliptical class proposed by Branco and Dey (2001). This subclass contains the entire family of normal independent distributions, also known as scale mixtures of normal distributions (SMN) (Lange and Sinsheimer 1993). In addition, the skew-normal and skewed versions of some other classical symmetric distributions are SMSN members: the skew-t (ST), the skew-slash (SSL), and the skew-contaminated normal (SCN), for example. These distributions have heavier tails than the typical normal one, and thus they seem to be a reasonable choice for robust inference. The proposed EM-type algorithm and methods are implemented in the R package mixsmsn.

In Chap. 1, we present a motivating example, where it seems that a better degree of explanation is obtained using mixtures of SMSN distributions than using symmetric components.

In Chap. 2, we present background material on mixture models and the EM algorithm for maximum likelihood estimation. This is followed by the derivation of the observed information matrix to obtain the standard errors.

In Chap. 3, for the sake of completeness, we define the multivariate SMSN distributions and study some of its important properties, viz., moments, kurtosis, linear transformations, marginal and conditional distributions, among others. Further, the EM algorithm for performing maximum likelihood estimation is presented.

In Chap. 4, we propose a finite mixture of univariate SMSN distributions (FM-SMSN) and an EM-type algorithm for maximum likelihood estimation. The associated observed information matrix is obtained analytically. The methodology proposed is illustrated considering the analysis of a real data set and simulation studies.

In Chap. 5, we consider a flexible class of models, with elements that are finite mixtures of multivariate SMSN distributions. A general EM-type algorithm is employed for iteratively computing parameter estimates and this is discussed with emphasis on finite mixtures of skew-normal, skew-t, skew-slash, and skew-contaminated normal distributions. Further, a general information-based method for approximating the asymptotic covariance matrix of the estimates is also presented.

Finally in Chap. 6, we present a proposal to deal with mixtures of regression models by assuming that the random errors follow scale mixtures of skew-normal distributions. This approach allows us to model data with great flexibility, accommodating skewness and heavy tails at the same time. A simple EM-type algorithm to perform maximum likelihood inference of the parameters of the proposed model is derived. A real data set is analyzed, illustrating the usefulness of the proposed method.

We hope that the publication of this text will enhance the spread of ideas that are currently trickling thought the literature of mixture models. The skew models and methods developed recently in this field have yet to reach their largest possible audience, partly because the results are scattered in various journals. Please send any comments to us at hlachos@uconn.edu, celsoromulo@gmail.com, or camila.zeller@ice.ufjf.br. Víctor H. Lachos was supported by CNPq-Brazil (BPPesq) and São Paulo State Research Foundation (FAPESP). Celso Rômulo Barbosa Cabral was supported by CNPq (BPPesq) and Amazonas State Research Foundation (FAPEAM, Universal project). Camila Borelli Zeller was supported by CNPq (BPPesq and Universal project) and Minas Gerais State Research Foundation (FAPEMIG, Universal project).

Storrs, USA — Víctor Hugo Lachos Dávila
Manaus, Brazil — Celso Rômulo Barbosa Cabral
Juiz de Fora, Brazil — Camila Borelli Zeller
January 2018

Contents

Chapter 1
Motivation

Modeling based on finite mixture distributions is a rapidly developing area with an exploding range of applications. Finite mixture models are nowadays applied in such diverse areas as biology, biometrics, genetics, medicine, and marketing, among others. There are various features of finite mixture distributions that make them useful in statistical modeling. For instance, statistical models which are based on finite mixture distributions capture many specific properties of real data such as multimodality, skewness, kurtosis, and unobserved heterogeneity. The importance of mixtures can be noted from the large number of books on the subject, like Lindsay (1995), Böhning (2000), McLachlan and Peel (2000), Frühwirth-Schnatter (2006), and Mengersen et al. (2011). See also the special edition of the journal *Computational Statistics & Data Analysis* (Böhning et al. 2014).

Formally speaking, given densities $g_j(\cdot)$ and weights $p_j \geq 0$, $j = 1, \ldots, G$, such that $\sum_{j=1}^{G} p_j = 1$, a *finite mixture of densities* is the density

$$f(\mathbf{y}) = \sum_{j=1}^{G} p_j g_j(\mathbf{y}), \quad \mathbf{y} \in \mathbb{R}^q. \tag{1.1}$$

The density $g_j(\cdot)$ is named the *jth component of the mixture.*

Finite mixtures are useful to model population heterogeneity, when we know that observations belong to G distinct subpopulations, but we do not know how to discriminate between them. As an example of unobserved heterogeneity in a population, consider the famous fishery data, which is freely available through the `R` package `bayesmix` (Gruen 2015). This data set has been analyzed by many authors see, for example, Titterington et al. (1985) and Frühwirth-Schnatter (2006). The data consists of 256 observations of fish lengths. Figure 1.1 presents the histogram of the data, and we can visualize several modes. Specialists agree that the source of the latent heterogeneity can be the age groups, which is a variable very hard to observe directly.

V. H. Lachos Dávila et al., *Finite Mixture of Skewed Distributions*,
SpringerBriefs in Statistics, https://doi.org/10.1007/978-3-319-98029-4_1

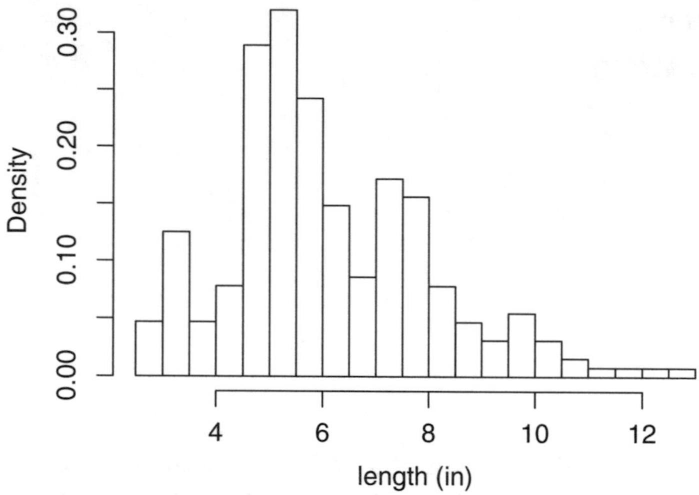

Fig. 1.1 Histogram of the fishery data

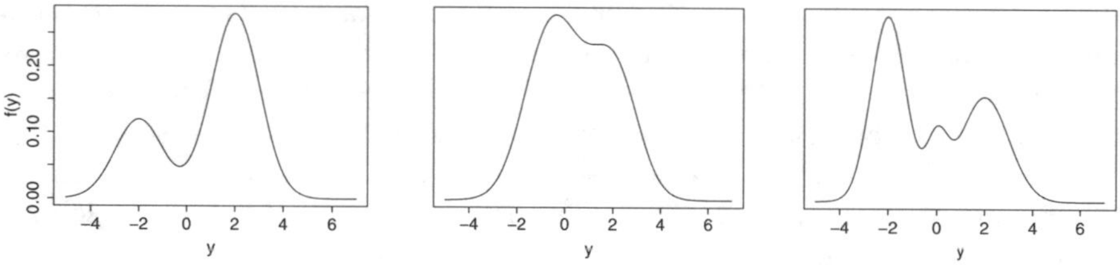

Fig. 1.2 Densities of mixtures of univariate normal distributions. Left: $\mu_1 = -2$, $\mu_2 = 2$, $\sigma_1^2 = \sigma_2^2 = 1$, $p_1 = 0.3$. Middle: $\mu_1 = -1$, $\mu_2 = 0$, $\mu_3 = 2$, $\sigma_1^2 = \sigma_2^2 = \sigma_3^2 = 1$, $p_1 = p_2 = 0.3$. Right: $\mu_1 = -2$, $\mu_2 = 0$, $\mu_3 = 2$, $\sigma_1^2 = 0.5$, $\sigma_2^2 = 0.2$, $\sigma_3^2 = 1$, $p_1 = 0.5$, $p_2 = 0.1$

Finite mixtures is also an extremely flexible class of distributions. To have a little idea of their capabilities, see Fig. 1.2, where we are considering mixtures of univariate normal distributions, given by $f(y) = \sum_{j=1}^{G} p_j \phi(y|\mu_j, \sigma_j^2)$, where $\phi(\cdot|\mu_j, \sigma_j^2)$ denotes the $\mathrm{N}(\mu_j, \sigma_j^2)$ density.

There is a formal mathematical motivation for using mixtures as such class of flexible probability models. The following theorem shows that any continuous density can be approximated by a proper finite mixture of *any* (not necessarily normal) continuous densities. See DasGupta (2008, Theorem 33.2) for more details.

Theorem 1.1 *Let $f(\cdot)$ and $g(\cdot)$ be continuous densities on $\mathbb{R}^q$. Given $\epsilon > 0$ and a compact set $C \subset \mathbb{R}^q$, there exists a finite mixture of the form $h(x) = \sum_{j=1}^{G} p_j \sigma_j^{-q} g\left((x - \mu_j)/\sigma_j\right)$ such that* $\sup_{x \in C} |f(x) - h(x)| < \epsilon$.

Observe that the theorem does not specify how many components G are necessary to approximate the density $f(\cdot)$.

Although mixtures of normal distributions have been applied during many years in several areas of knowledge to model data with a distribution having a complex structure, deviations from the normal assumption among the subpopulations, like strong asymmetry or heavy tails, are not uncommon. Sometimes these departures are not well captured by a finite mixture of normal distributions, or even by a finite mixture of a more robust symmetric distribution, like the Student-t. The main proposal of this book is to consider finite mixtures of distributions which belong to a family much more flexible than the normal or Student-t ones, allowing us to accommodate at the same time skewness, outliers and multimodality, besides achieving a more parsimonious model, because we expect that fewer components would be necessary to obtain the same degree of explanation obtained using normal, Student t, or other symmetric components.

As an example, consider the Body Mass Index (BMI) Data, which is freely available through the `R` package `mixsmsn` (Prates et al. 2013). Figure 1.3 shows a histogram of the data. We fitted some finite mixtures of normal and Student-t distributions to these data, with 2 and 3 components. To do so, we used the package `mixsmsn`. More details about the estimation process will be discussed in Chaps. 2 and 3.

Table 1.1 shows the values of the AIC (Akaike 1974) and BIC (Schwarz 1978) model selection criteria. When comparing several models, a specific criterion favors the model with the smallest criterion value. Besides the normal and Student-t models, we used as components some extensions of these distributions, namely the skew-normal and the skew-t ones. These distributions extend theirs, symmetric counterparts by the introduction of an additional parameter regulating skewness. More details about these models will be given in Chap. 3. From Table 1.1 we can see that the two criteria chose the models in the following order, from the best to the poorest: skew-t (2), normal (3), Student-t (3), Skew-normal (2), Student-t (2),

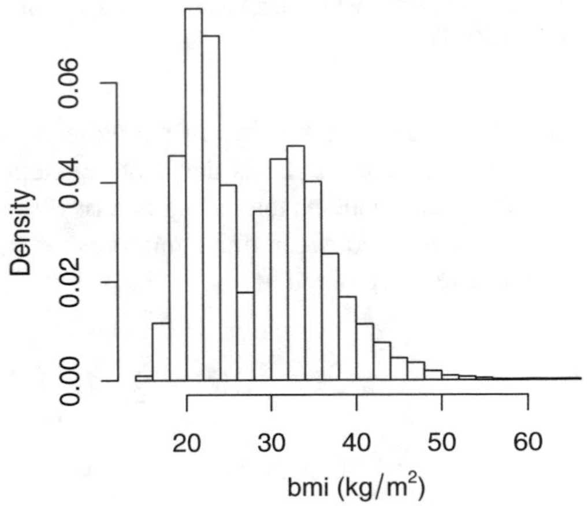

Fig. 1.3 Histogram of the BMI data

Table 1.1 BMI data

Model	BIC	AIC
Normal (2)	13,861.78	13,833.51
Normal (3)	13,787.05	13,741.83
Student-t (2)	13,814.37	13,786.10
Student-t (3)	13,787.51	13,742.29
Skew-normal (2)	13,803.36	13,763.79
Skew-t (2)	13,777.13	13,737.56

BIC criterion for several mixture models. The number in parenthesis denotes the number of components

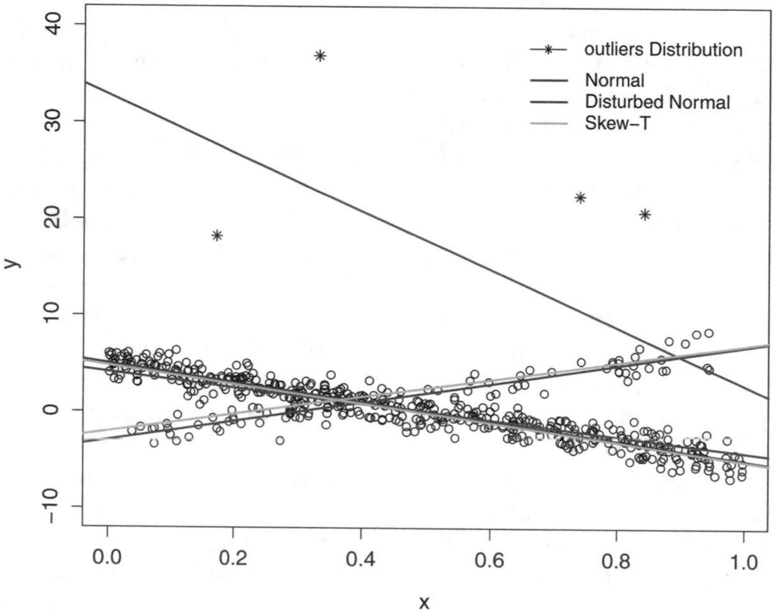

Fig. 1.4 Contaminated normal mixture regression model. Normal and Student-t mixture regression models fit

and normal (2)—the number in parenthesis denotes the number of components. From these results, it seems that a better degree of explanation is obtained using two skew-t components than using two or three normal or Student-t components.

We can also consider finite mixtures of regression models. In the univariate normal case it is defined as

$$f(y|\boldsymbol{\theta}) = \sum_{j=1}^{G} p_j \phi\big(y|\mathbf{x}^\top \boldsymbol{\beta}_j, \sigma_j^2\big), \tag{1.2}$$

where $\mathbf{x}$ is a vector of covariates or explanatory variables and $\boldsymbol{\beta}_j$ is a vector of component-specific unknown regression coefficients. In Fig. 1.4, we depict a sample $y_i,\ i = 1, \ldots, 500$, from a finite mixture of normal regression models with $G = 2$, $\mathbf{x}_i^\top = (1, x_i)$, such that $x_i \sim \mathrm{U}(0, 1)$, with the following setup: $\boldsymbol{\beta}_1 = (\beta_{01}, \beta_{11})^\top = (5, -10)^\top$, $\boldsymbol{\beta}_2 = (\beta_{02}, \beta_{12})^\top = (-3, 10)^\top, \sigma_1^2 = \sigma_2^2 = 1$ and $p_1 = 0.8$. Then we fitted the correct model, which corresponds to the red lines in the figure. After this, we contaminated the sample, by replacing the observations y_{50}, y_{150}, y_{250}, and y_{350} with the contaminated values $y_{50}^* = y_{50} + 25$, $y_{150}^* = y_{150} + 15$, $y_{250}^* = y_{250} + 35$ and $y_{350}^* = y_{350} + 15$. Then we fitted the model again. This new fit is identified as the *disturbed model* in the figure (blue lines). Finally, we fitted a model where the normal distribution in (1.2) is replaced by the skew-t distribution (green lines). We can see that after contamination, the normal fit is strongly affected by the presence of outliers, which does not occur with the skew-t model.

Chapter 2
Maximum Likelihood Estimation in Normal Mixtures

At the beginning, the research on estimation of the parameters in finite mixture models was more focused in the normal components case. The first papers were published more than 100 years ago, as one of the first works in finite mixtures that come to our notice is Pearson (1894), who used the method of moments to fit a mixture of two normal components to the crabs data (Weldon 1893). Several works based on the method of moments followed the Pearson's one. Among them, Charlier and Wicksell (1924), Doetsch (1928) and Strömgren (1934). Rao (1948) was the first author to propose maximum likelihood (ML) estimation in finite mixtures of normal distributions, although his solution was restricted to the two components case. In the multivariate case, Wolfe (1965, 1967) also proposed ML estimation, and extended his results to cluster analysis. ML estimation in the case of a finite mixture of G components with equal variances was explored by Hasselblad (1966), who extended his results to exponential families in Hasselblad (1969). But the major breakthrough concerned with ML estimation in finite mixtures was the paper of Dempster et al. (1977), which established the theoretical basis of a whole line of research using the EM algorithm. After this, the research in finite mixtures exploded and it is almost impossible to provide an exhaustive list of references. The book of McLachlan and Peel (2000) provides a good review of the work in this area up to its publication. Important references also are the special volumes Böhning and Seidel (2003), and Böhning et al. (2007, 2014).

In this chapter we review the general theory of ML estimation in finite mixture models using the EM algorithm, with application in the model with multivariate normal components.

V. H. Lachos Dávila et al., *Finite Mixture of Skewed Distributions*,
SpringerBriefs in Statistics, https://doi.org/10.1007/978-3-319-98029-4_2

2.1 EM Algorithm for Finite Mixtures

In what follows we consider a random sample $\mathbf{Y}_1, \ldots, \mathbf{Y}_n$ from the mixture model (1.1). Hereafter, we assume that $g_j(\cdot) = g(\cdot|\boldsymbol{\theta}_j)$, $j = 1, \ldots, G$. That is, the densities $g_j(\cdot)$ belong to the same parametric family.

A useful interpretation of the finite mixture model is consequence of the following representation: let $\mathbf{Z}_i = (Z_{i1}, \ldots, Z_{iG})$, such that

$$P(Z_{ij} = 1) = p_j, \quad \text{and} \quad \mathbf{Y}_i|Z_{ij} = 1 \sim g(\cdot|\boldsymbol{\theta}_j). \tag{2.1}$$

If $Z_{ij} = 1$, then $Z_{ik} = 0$ for $k \neq j$. $\mathbf{Z}_i$ is known as the *allocation vector*. $\mathbf{Z}_i$ has only one element different from zero. If this element is in the jth position of the vector $\mathbf{Z}_i$, then $\mathbf{Y}_i$ is allocated to subpopulation j. The distribution of the vector $\mathbf{Z}_i$ is multinomial with one trial and probabilities $p_1, \ldots, p_G$, and we use the notation $\mathbf{Z}_i \sim \text{Multinomial}(1; p_1, \ldots, p_G)$. It is straightforward to prove that marginally $\mathbf{Y}_i$ has density (1.1), to be more specific,

$$f(\mathbf{y}_i|\boldsymbol{\theta}) = \sum_{j=1}^{G} p_j g(\mathbf{y}_i|\boldsymbol{\theta}_j), \quad \mathbf{y}_i \in \mathbb{R}^q$$

where $\boldsymbol{\theta} = (\boldsymbol{\theta}_1^\top, \ldots, \boldsymbol{\theta}_G^\top, p_1, \ldots, p_G)^\top$ is the vector with all parameters in the model. Using lowercase letters to denote observed values, the likelihood function associated with the sample $\mathbf{y} = (\mathbf{y}_1^\top, \ldots, \mathbf{y}_n^\top)^\top$ is given by

$$L(\boldsymbol{\theta}|\mathbf{y}) = \prod_{i=1}^{n} \sum_{j=1}^{G} p_j g(\mathbf{y}_i|\boldsymbol{\theta}_j).$$

Direct maximization of $L(\cdot|\mathbf{y})$ can lead to a difficult and unstable numerical problem. Instead, the best option is to use the EM algorithm of Dempster et al. (1977).

To develop the algorithm, we use a data augmentation framework based on representation (2.1). Let $\mathbf{z} = (\mathbf{z}_1^\top, \ldots, \mathbf{z}_n^\top)^\top$. The *complete-data likelihood* is the likelihood function obtained as if $(\mathbf{y}^\top, \mathbf{z}^\top)^\top$ were observable, that is,

$$\ell_c(\boldsymbol{\theta}|\mathbf{y}, \mathbf{z}) = \prod_{i=1}^{n} \pi(\mathbf{y}|\mathbf{z})\pi(\mathbf{z}) = \prod_{i=1}^{n} \prod_{j=1}^{G} g(\mathbf{y}_i|\boldsymbol{\theta}_j)^{z_{ij}} p_j^{z_{ij}}, \tag{2.2}$$

where $\pi(\mathbf{z})$ denotes the density of $\mathbf{Z}$ and $\pi(\mathbf{y}|\mathbf{z})$ denotes the conditional density of $\mathbf{Y}|\mathbf{Z} = \mathbf{z}$.

Now we proceed by implementing the two steps of the EM algorithm: the E-step (expectation) and the M-step (maximization). For more details about the algorithm and its applications in mixture models, see McLachlan and Krishnan (2008). In what follows $\widehat{\boldsymbol{\theta}}^{(k)}$ indicates the estimate of $\boldsymbol{\theta}$ at stage k of the algorithm. The E-step consists in taking the conditional expectation

$$Q\left(\boldsymbol{\theta}|\widehat{\boldsymbol{\theta}}^{(k)}\right) = \mathrm{E}\left[\log \ell_c(\boldsymbol{\theta}|\mathbf{y},\mathbf{z})|\mathbf{y},\widehat{\boldsymbol{\theta}}^{(k)}\right],$$

where the expectation is being affected using $\widehat{\boldsymbol{\theta}}^{(k)}$ for $\boldsymbol{\theta}$—this is the so-called Q-*function*. Now, observe that

$$\mathrm{E}\left[\log \ell_c(\boldsymbol{\theta}|\mathbf{y},\mathbf{z})|\mathbf{y},\widehat{\boldsymbol{\theta}}^{(k)}\right] = \mathrm{E}\left\{\sum_{i=1}^{n}\sum_{j=1}^{G} Z_{ij}\left[\log g(\mathbf{y}_i|\boldsymbol{\theta}_j) + \log p_j\right]|\mathbf{y},\widehat{\boldsymbol{\theta}}^{(k)}\right\} \tag{2.3}$$

$$= \sum_{i=1}^{n}\sum_{j=1}^{G} \mathrm{E}\left(Z_{ij}|\mathbf{y},\widehat{\boldsymbol{\theta}}^{(k)}\right)\left[\log g(\mathbf{y}_i|\boldsymbol{\theta}_j) + \log p_j\right]. \tag{2.4}$$

Observe that it is easy to compute $\mathrm{E}(Z_{ij}|\mathbf{y},\widehat{\boldsymbol{\theta}}^{(k)})$, because the distribution of Z_{ij} is Bernoulli with probability of success p_j. Then,

$$\widehat{z}_{ij}^{(k+1)} \equiv \mathrm{E}\left(Z_{ij}|\mathbf{y},\widehat{\boldsymbol{\theta}}^{(k)}\right) = P\left(Z_{ij}=1|\mathbf{y},\widehat{\boldsymbol{\theta}}^{(k)}\right) \propto g\left(\mathbf{y}_i|\widehat{\boldsymbol{\theta}}_j^{(k)}\right)\widehat{p}_j^{(k)},$$

implying that

$$z_{ij}^{(k+1)} = \frac{g\left(\mathbf{y}_i|\widehat{\boldsymbol{\theta}}_j^{(k)}\right)\widehat{p}_j^{(k)}}{\sum_{m=1}^{G} g\left(\mathbf{y}_i|\widehat{\boldsymbol{\theta}}_m^{(k)}\right)\widehat{p}_m^{(k)}}, \quad j = 1,\ldots,G.$$

The M-step consists in to maximize the Q-function (2.4). Regarding the parameters p_j, $j = 1,\ldots,G$, this is equivalent to maximize the function

$$\sum_{i=1}^{n}\sum_{j=1}^{G} \widehat{z}_{ij}^{(k+1)} \log p_j$$

with respect to p_j, $j = 1,\ldots,G$. Then, it is straightforward to prove that

$$\widehat{p}_j^{(k+1)} = \frac{1}{n}\sum_{i=1}^{n} \widehat{z}_{ij}^{(k+1)}.$$

Until now we have not considered as components a specific parametric family of distributions. To illustrate the theory, let us assume that we have a mixture density with a normal q-variate jth component $\mathrm{N}_q(\boldsymbol{\mu}_j, \boldsymbol{\Sigma}_j)$ with weight p_j, where $\boldsymbol{\mu}_j$ and $\boldsymbol{\Sigma}_j$ are the mean vector and the covariance matrix, respectively, $j = 1, \ldots, G$. Then, we can see that the M-step is equivalent to maximize the function

$$\sum_{i=1}^{n}\sum_{j=1}^{G} \widehat{z}_{ij}^{(k+1)} \log \phi_q(\mathbf{y}_i|\boldsymbol{\mu}_j, \boldsymbol{\Sigma}_j)$$

with respect to $\boldsymbol{\mu}_j$ and $\boldsymbol{\Sigma}_j$, where $\phi_q(\mathbf{y}_i|\boldsymbol{\mu}_j, \boldsymbol{\Sigma}_j)$ is the $\mathrm{N}_q(\boldsymbol{\mu}_j, \boldsymbol{\Sigma}_j)$ density. But, for fixed j, this is equivalent to maximize the normal weighted log-likelihood function

$$\sum_{i=1}^{n} \widehat{z}_{ij}^{(k+1)} \log \phi_q(\mathbf{y}_i|\boldsymbol{\mu}_j, \boldsymbol{\Sigma}_j).$$

This problem has a well-known solution given by

$$\widehat{\boldsymbol{\mu}}_j^{(k+1)} = \frac{\sum_{i=1}^{n} \widehat{z}_{ij}^{(k+1)} \mathbf{y}_i}{\sum_{i=1}^{n} \widehat{z}_{ij}^{(k+1)}}, \quad \text{and}$$

$$\widehat{\boldsymbol{\Sigma}}_j^{(k+1)} = \frac{\sum_{i=1}^{n} \widehat{z}_{ij}^{(k+1)} \left(\mathbf{y}_i - \widehat{\boldsymbol{\mu}}_i^{(k+1)}\right)\left(\mathbf{y}_i - \widehat{\boldsymbol{\mu}}_i^{(k+1)}\right)^\top}{\sum_{i=1}^{n} \widehat{z}_{ij}^{(k)}}, \quad j = 1, \ldots, G.$$

2.2 Standard Errors

In this section we explain how to obtain standard errors estimates for the EM estimators. First, we review some basic concepts. For more details, see Lehmann (1999, Sec 7.5). Let $\mathbf{Y} = (\mathbf{Y}_1^\top, \ldots, \mathbf{Y}_n^\top)^\top$ be a random sample from $f(\cdot|\boldsymbol{\theta})$. For regular models, the expected information matrix is defined as

$$I(\boldsymbol{\theta}) = \mathrm{E}\left[\frac{\partial \log f(\mathbf{Y}_1|\boldsymbol{\theta})}{\partial \boldsymbol{\theta}} \left(\frac{\partial \log f(\mathbf{Y}_1|\boldsymbol{\theta})}{\partial \boldsymbol{\theta}}\right)^\top |\boldsymbol{\theta}\right]. \tag{2.5}$$

Under suitable regularity conditions, it is possible to prove that

$$I(\boldsymbol{\theta}) = -\mathrm{E}\left[\frac{\partial^2 \log f(\mathbf{Y}_1|\boldsymbol{\theta})}{\partial \boldsymbol{\theta} \partial \boldsymbol{\theta}^\top} |\boldsymbol{\theta}\right],$$

that is, the negative of expectation of the hessian matrix.

Let $\widehat{\boldsymbol{\theta}}$ be the maximum likelihood estimator (MLE) of $\boldsymbol{\theta}$. Under regularity conditions, the asymptotic covariance matrix of $\widehat{\boldsymbol{\theta}}$ is $I(\boldsymbol{\theta})^{-1}/n$. This matrix depends on the unknown parameter $\boldsymbol{\theta}$, and is useless for inference. But, under suitable conditions, the MLE is consistent and, in general, $I(\widehat{\boldsymbol{\theta}})^{-1}$ is a consistent estimator of $I(\boldsymbol{\theta})^{-1}$.

In practice, for complex models, it is not possible, or it is very difficult, to obtain the expected information matrix. An alternative is to approximate it using the so-called observed information matrix, which is defined to be

$$\mathbf{J}_o(\widehat{\boldsymbol{\theta}}|\mathbf{Y}) = -\frac{1}{n}\sum_{i=1}^{n}\frac{\partial^2 \log f(\mathbf{Y}_i|\boldsymbol{\theta})}{\partial\boldsymbol{\theta}\partial\boldsymbol{\theta}^\top}\Big|_{\boldsymbol{\theta}=\widehat{\boldsymbol{\theta}}} .$$

By the strong law of large numbers,

$$\mathbf{J}_o(\widehat{\boldsymbol{\theta}}|\mathbf{Y}) \to I(\boldsymbol{\theta})$$

when $n \to \infty$, almost surely. So, for large n, it is reasonable to use

$$\frac{\mathbf{J}_o(\widehat{\boldsymbol{\theta}}|\mathbf{Y})^{-1}}{n} = \left(-\sum_{i=1}^{n}\frac{\partial^2 \log f(\mathbf{Y}_i|\boldsymbol{\theta})}{\partial\boldsymbol{\theta}\partial\boldsymbol{\theta}^\top}\Big|_{\boldsymbol{\theta}=\widehat{\boldsymbol{\theta}}}\right)^{-1} \tag{2.6}$$

as an approximation of the asymptotic covariance matrix of $\widehat{\boldsymbol{\theta}}$.

An alternative is the following. By (2.5) and the strong law of large numbers,

$$\frac{1}{n}\sum_{i=1}^{n}\frac{\partial \log f(\mathbf{Y}_i|\boldsymbol{\theta})}{\partial\boldsymbol{\theta}}\left(\frac{\partial \log f(\mathbf{Y}_i|\boldsymbol{\theta})}{\partial\boldsymbol{\theta}}\right)^\top\Big|_{\boldsymbol{\theta}=\widehat{\boldsymbol{\theta}}} \to I(\boldsymbol{\theta})$$

when $n \to \infty$, almost surely. That is, the asymptotic covariance matrix of $\widehat{\boldsymbol{\theta}}$ can be approximated by

$$\left[\sum_{i=1}^{n}\frac{\partial \log f(\mathbf{Y}_i|\boldsymbol{\theta})}{\partial\boldsymbol{\theta}}\left(\frac{\partial \log f(\mathbf{Y}_i|\boldsymbol{\theta})}{\partial\boldsymbol{\theta}}\right)^\top\Big|_{\boldsymbol{\theta}=\widehat{\boldsymbol{\theta}}}\right]^{-1} . \tag{2.7}$$

Consider the complete-data likelihood given in (2.2). It is possible to show, see McLachlan and Peel (2000, p. 66), that

$$\frac{\partial \log f(\mathbf{y}_i|\boldsymbol{\theta})}{\partial\boldsymbol{\theta}} = \mathrm{E}\left[\frac{\partial \log \ell_c(\boldsymbol{\theta}|\mathbf{y}_i, \mathbf{z}_i)}{\partial\boldsymbol{\theta}}|\mathbf{y}, \boldsymbol{\theta}\right], \tag{2.8}$$

where $\ell_c(\boldsymbol{\theta}|\mathbf{y}_i, \mathbf{z}_i)$ is the complete-data likelihood formed from the single "observation" $(\mathbf{y}_i, \mathbf{z}_i)$, $i = 1, \ldots, n$. Formulas (2.7) and (2.8) imply that the asymptotic covariance matrix of $\widehat{\boldsymbol{\theta}}$ can be approximated by

$$\left\{\sum_{i=1}^{n} \mathrm{E}\left[\frac{\partial \log \ell_c(\boldsymbol{\theta}|\mathbf{y}_i, \mathbf{z}_i)}{\partial \boldsymbol{\theta}} |\mathbf{y}, \boldsymbol{\theta}\right] |_{\theta=\widehat{\theta}} \mathrm{E}\left[\frac{\partial \log \ell_c(\boldsymbol{\theta}|\mathbf{y}_i, \mathbf{z}_i)}{\partial \boldsymbol{\theta}} |\mathbf{y}, \boldsymbol{\theta}\right]^{\top} |_{\theta=\widehat{\theta}}\right\}^{-1}.$$

For finite mixture models we have, from (2.2),

$$\log \ell_c(\boldsymbol{\theta}|\mathbf{y}_i, \mathbf{z}_i) = \sum_{j=1}^{G} z_{ij}[\log f(\mathbf{y}_i|\boldsymbol{\theta}_j) + \log p_j].$$

Then,

$$\begin{aligned}
\mathrm{E}\left[\frac{\partial \log \ell_c(\boldsymbol{\theta}|\mathbf{y}_i, \mathbf{z}_i)}{\partial \boldsymbol{\theta}} |\mathbf{y}, \boldsymbol{\theta}\right] &= \mathrm{E}\left\{\sum_{j=1}^{G} Z_{ij} \left[\frac{\partial(\log f(\mathbf{y}_i|\boldsymbol{\theta}_j) + \log p_j)}{\partial \boldsymbol{\theta}}\right] |\mathbf{y}, \boldsymbol{\theta}\right\} \\
&= \sum_{j=1}^{G} \mathrm{E}(Z_{ij}|\mathbf{y}, \boldsymbol{\theta}) \left[\frac{\partial(\log f(\mathbf{y}_i|\boldsymbol{\theta}_j) + \log p_j)}{\partial \boldsymbol{\theta}}\right].
\end{aligned}$$

As an example, let us consider the normal mixture case, in which the jth component is $\mathrm{N}_q(\boldsymbol{\mu}_j, \boldsymbol{\Sigma}_j)$, $j = 1, \ldots, G$. Let us define $\mathbf{p} = (p_1, \ldots, p_{G-1})^{\top}$ and $\boldsymbol{\omega}_j$ a vector containing the $q(1+q)/2$ distinct elements of $\boldsymbol{\Sigma}_j$, $j = 1, \ldots, G$. Then, the vector with all parameters in the model can be written as

$$\boldsymbol{\theta} = \left(\mathbf{p}^{\top}, \boldsymbol{\mu}_1^{\top}, \ldots, \boldsymbol{\mu}_G^{\top}, \boldsymbol{\omega}_1^{\top}, \ldots, \boldsymbol{\omega}_G^{\top}\right)^{\top},$$

and partitioning accordingly

$$\sum_{j=1}^{G} \widehat{z}_{ij} \frac{\partial(\log \phi_q(\mathbf{y}_i|\boldsymbol{\mu}_j, \boldsymbol{\Sigma}_j) + \log p_j)}{\partial \boldsymbol{\theta}} |_{\theta=\widehat{\theta}} \equiv \left(\widehat{\mathbf{s}}_{\mathbf{p}_i}^{\top}, \widehat{\mathbf{s}}_{\mu_{1i}}^{\top}, \ldots, \widehat{\mathbf{s}}_{\mu_{Gi}}^{\top}, \widehat{\mathbf{s}}_{\omega_{1i}}^{\top}, \ldots, \widehat{\mathbf{s}}_{\omega_{Gi}}^{\top}\right)^{\top},$$

where $\widehat{z}_{ij}$ is $\mathrm{E}(Z_{ij}|\mathbf{y}, \boldsymbol{\theta})$ evaluated at $\widehat{\boldsymbol{\theta}}$, that is,

$$\widehat{z}_{ij} = \frac{\phi_q(\mathbf{y}_i|\widehat{\boldsymbol{\mu}}_j, \widehat{\boldsymbol{\Sigma}}_j)\widehat{p}_j}{\sum_{m=1}^{G} \phi_q(\mathbf{y}_i|\widehat{\boldsymbol{\mu}}_m, \widehat{\boldsymbol{\Sigma}}_m)\widehat{p}_m}$$

and

$$\begin{aligned}
\widehat{\mathbf{s}}_{\mathbf{p}_i} &= \sum_{j=1}^{G} \widehat{z}_{ij} \frac{\partial(\log \phi_q(\mathbf{y}_i|\boldsymbol{\mu}_j, \boldsymbol{\Sigma}_j) + \log p_j)}{\partial \mathbf{p}} |_{\theta=\widehat{\theta}} \\
\widehat{\mathbf{s}}_{\mu_{ji}} &= \widehat{z}_{ij} \frac{\partial(\log \phi_q(\mathbf{y}_i|\boldsymbol{\mu}_j, \boldsymbol{\Sigma}_j) + \log p_j)}{\partial \boldsymbol{\mu}_j} |_{\theta=\widehat{\theta}}
\end{aligned}$$

$$\widehat{\mathbf{s}}_{\omega_{ji}} = \widehat{z}_{ij} \frac{\partial(\log \phi_q(\mathbf{y}_i|\boldsymbol{\mu}_j, \boldsymbol{\Sigma}_j) + \log p_j)}{\partial \boldsymbol{\omega}_j}\Big|_{\theta=\widehat{\theta}}, \qquad i = 1, \ldots, n.$$

For fixed i, it is straightforward to show that the jth element of the vector $\widehat{\mathbf{s}}_{\mathbf{p}_i}$ is given by

$$\left(\widehat{\mathbf{s}}_{\mathbf{p}_i}\right)_j = \frac{\widehat{z}_{ij}}{p_j} - \frac{\widehat{z}_{iG}}{p_G}, \qquad j = 1, \ldots, G-1.$$

Using matrix differentiation, we can prove that

$$\widehat{\mathbf{s}}_{\boldsymbol{\mu}_{ji}} = \widehat{z}_{ij} \widehat{\boldsymbol{\Sigma}}_j^{-1} (\mathbf{y}_i - \widehat{\boldsymbol{\mu}}_j), \qquad j = 1, \ldots, G,$$

and

$$\left(\widehat{\mathbf{s}}_{\omega_{ji}}\right)_h = \frac{1}{2} \widehat{z}_{ij} (2 - \delta_{rs}) \left[-\left(\widehat{\boldsymbol{\Sigma}}_j^{-1}\right)_{rs} + (\mathbf{y}_i - \widehat{\mu}_j)^\top \widehat{\sigma}_j^{(r)} (\mathbf{y}_i - \widehat{\mu}_j)^\top \widehat{\sigma}_j^{(s)} \right],$$

where δ_{rs} is the Kronecker delta, the hth element of $\widehat{\mathbf{s}}_{\omega_{ji}}$ corresponds to the (r, s)th element of $\boldsymbol{\Sigma}_j$ and where $\widehat{\sigma}_j^{(r)}$ is the rth column of $\widehat{\boldsymbol{\Sigma}}_j^{-1}$, $j = 1, \ldots, G$. See McLachlan and Basford (1988, p. 48) for more details.

Chapter 3
Scale Mixtures of Skew-Normal Distributions

Andrews and Mallows (1974) discussed a class of robust distributions as scale mixtures of normal (SMN) distributions, which contains a group of thick-tailed distributions. Their work was extended by Branco and Dey (2001), introducing the class of scale mixtures of skew-normal (SMSN) distributions, which includes the former class by the introduction of a parameter regulating skewness. In this chapter, we discuss some properties of the SMSN distributions in the multivariate setting. The main virtue of the members of this family is that they are easy to simulate from and they also lend themselves to an EM-type algorithm for maximum likelihood estimation. Results obtained from simulated and a real data set are reported illustrating the usefulness of the proposed distributions.

3.1 Introduction

A normal distribution is a routine assumption for analyzing real data, but it may be unrealistic, specially for data with strong skewness and heavy tails. In practice, there are a great number of skewed or heavy-tailed data, for instance, data on family income, CD4 count data from AIDS studies, etc. Thus, one need to develop a flexible class of models that can readily adapt to the non-normality behavior of the data. Flexible models that include several known distributions, including the normal distribution are of particular importance, since such models can adapt to distributions that are in the neighborhood of the normal model. Andrews and Mallows (1974) developed the class of scale mixtures of normal (SMN) distributions, which contains a group of thick-tailed distributions that are often used for robust inference of symmetrical data. In this chapter, we further generalize the SMN class of distributions and combine skewness with heavy tails. This class of distributions is attractive as it simultaneously models skewness and heavy tails, it

V. H. Lachos Dávila et al., *Finite Mixture of Skewed Distributions*,
SpringerBriefs in Statistics, https://doi.org/10.1007/978-3-319-98029-4_3

has a stochastic representation for easy implementation of the EM algorithm, and also facilitates the study of many useful properties.

The skew-normal (SN) distribution extends the normal one by allowing a shape parameter to account for skewness. Azzalini (1985) proposed a univariate form, which was generalized to the multivariate case by Azzalini and Dalla-Valle (1996). According to their definition, we say that a p-dimensional random vector $\mathbf{Y}$ has a skew-normal distribution with location vector $\boldsymbol{\mu}$, scale matrix $\boldsymbol{\Sigma}$, and shape parameter vector $\boldsymbol{\lambda}$ when it has probability density function (pdf)

$$f(\mathbf{y}) = 2\phi_p(\mathbf{y}|\boldsymbol{\mu}, \boldsymbol{\Sigma})\Phi\big(\boldsymbol{\lambda}^\top\boldsymbol{\sigma}^{-1}(\mathbf{y} - \boldsymbol{\mu})\big), \quad \mathbf{y} \in \mathbb{R}^p, \tag{3.1}$$

where $\Phi(\cdot)$ is the cumulative distribution function (cdf) of the standard normal distribution, $\boldsymbol{\sigma}$ is a diagonal matrix formed by the standard deviations of a covariance matrix $\boldsymbol{\Sigma}$, such that $\boldsymbol{\Sigma} = \boldsymbol{\sigma}\overline{\boldsymbol{\Sigma}}\boldsymbol{\sigma}$, where $\overline{\boldsymbol{\Sigma}}$ is a correlation matrix. When $\boldsymbol{\lambda} = \mathbf{0}$, the SN distribution reduces to the normal distribution.

The SN distribution has the following alternative representation: consider the random vector

$$\begin{pmatrix} T_o \\ \mathbf{T}_1 \end{pmatrix} \sim \mathrm{N}_{1+p}\left[\mathbf{0}, \begin{pmatrix} 1 & \boldsymbol{\delta}^\top \\ \boldsymbol{\delta} & \overline{\boldsymbol{\Sigma}} \end{pmatrix}\right], \tag{3.2}$$

where $\boldsymbol{\delta} = \overline{\boldsymbol{\Sigma}}\boldsymbol{\lambda}/(1 + \boldsymbol{\lambda}^\top\overline{\boldsymbol{\Sigma}}\boldsymbol{\lambda})^{1/2}$. Then, it is straightforward to show that the distribution of $\mathbf{Z} = (\mathbf{T}_1|T_0 > 0)$ is $f(\mathbf{z}) = 2\phi_p(\mathbf{z}|\mathbf{0}, \overline{\boldsymbol{\Sigma}})\Phi(\boldsymbol{\lambda}^\top\mathbf{z})$. To incorporate a location $\boldsymbol{\mu} \in \mathbb{R}^p$ and a positive definite scale matrix $\boldsymbol{\Sigma}$, we define $\mathbf{Y} = \boldsymbol{\mu} + \boldsymbol{\sigma}\mathbf{Z}$. Then, $\mathbf{Y}$ has the distribution defined in (3.1).

Hereafter we consider a variant form of the SN distribution of Azzalini and Dalla-Valle (1996). First, we replace the correlation matrix $\overline{\boldsymbol{\Sigma}}$ in (3.2) with the identity matrix $\mathbf{I}_p$. Then, the SN is defined as the distribution of the vector $\mathbf{Y} = \boldsymbol{\mu} + \boldsymbol{\Sigma}^{1/2}\mathbf{Z}$, where $\mathbf{Z} = (\mathbf{T}_1|T_0 > 0)$ and $\boldsymbol{\Sigma}^{1/2}$ is a square root of a positive definite matrix. This square root can be defined using the spectral decomposition of $\boldsymbol{\Sigma}$, see Gentle (2007, Sec. 3.8.8), for example. The resulting pdf is

$$f(\mathbf{y}) = 2\phi_p(\mathbf{y}|\boldsymbol{\mu}, \boldsymbol{\Sigma})\Phi\big(\boldsymbol{\lambda}^\top\boldsymbol{\Sigma}^{-1/2}(\mathbf{y} - \boldsymbol{\mu})\big), \quad \mathbf{y} \in \mathbb{R}^p.$$

We use the notation $\mathbf{Y} \sim \mathrm{SN}_p(\boldsymbol{\mu}, \boldsymbol{\Sigma}, \boldsymbol{\lambda})$.

Let $\mathbf{Z} = (\mathbf{T}_1|T_0 > 0)$ having an SN distribution, where T_0 and $\mathbf{T}_1$ are defined in (3.2) with $\overline{\boldsymbol{\Sigma}} = \mathbf{I}_p$. We can write

$$\begin{pmatrix} T_o \\ \mathbf{T}_1 \end{pmatrix} \overset{d}{=} \begin{pmatrix} X_0 \\ \boldsymbol{\delta}X_0 + (\mathbf{I}_p - \boldsymbol{\delta}\boldsymbol{\delta}^\top)^{1/2}\mathbf{X}_1 \end{pmatrix},$$

where $X_0 \sim \mathrm{N}(0, 1)$ and $\mathbf{X}_1 \sim \mathrm{N}_p(\mathbf{0}, \mathbf{I})$ are independent and "$\overset{d}{=}$" means that the random vectors have the same distribution. Using this fact and Theorem 3.1

of Arellano-Valle et al. (2002), we have that $\mathbf{Z} \stackrel{d}{=} \boldsymbol{\delta}|X_0| + (\mathbf{I}_p - \boldsymbol{\delta}\boldsymbol{\delta}^\top)^{1/2}\mathbf{X}_1$. Thus, a stochastic representation of $\mathbf{Y} \sim \mathrm{SN}_p(\boldsymbol{\mu}, \boldsymbol{\Sigma}, \boldsymbol{\lambda})$, which can be used to derive several of its properties, is given by

$$\mathbf{Y} \stackrel{d}{=} \boldsymbol{\mu} + \boldsymbol{\Sigma}^{1/2}\left(\boldsymbol{\delta}|X_0| + \left(\mathbf{I}_p - \boldsymbol{\delta}\boldsymbol{\delta}^\top\right)^{1/2}\mathbf{X}_1\right), \quad \text{with} \quad \boldsymbol{\delta} = \frac{\boldsymbol{\lambda}}{\sqrt{1+\boldsymbol{\lambda}^\top\boldsymbol{\lambda}}}. \tag{3.3}$$

Using the result above and the fact that $|X_0|$ follows a half-normal distribution with expectation $(2/\pi)^{1/2}$ and variance $1 - 2/\pi$, we have that the expectation and the covariance matrix of $\mathbf{Y}$ are given, respectively, by

$$\mathrm{E}[\mathbf{Y}] = \boldsymbol{\mu} + \sqrt{\frac{2}{\pi}}\boldsymbol{\Sigma}^{1/2}\boldsymbol{\delta} \ \text{ and } \ \mathrm{Var}[\mathbf{Y}] = \boldsymbol{\Sigma} - \frac{2}{\pi}\boldsymbol{\Sigma}^{1/2}\boldsymbol{\delta}\boldsymbol{\delta}^\top\boldsymbol{\Sigma}^{1/2}.$$

The moment generating function (mgf) of $\mathbf{Y} \sim \mathrm{SN}_p(\boldsymbol{\mu}, \boldsymbol{\Sigma}, \boldsymbol{\lambda})$ can be obtained with a small modification of the argument in Azzalini and Dalla-Valle (1996, eqn. 2.13). We find

$$\mathrm{M}_{\mathbf{y}}(\mathbf{s}) = 2e^{\mathbf{s}^\top\boldsymbol{\mu} + \frac{1}{2}\mathbf{s}^\top\boldsymbol{\Sigma}\mathbf{s}}\Phi\left(\boldsymbol{\delta}^\top\boldsymbol{\Sigma}^{1/2}\mathbf{s}\right). \tag{3.4}$$

Several extensions of the above model have been proposed, viz., the skew-t distribution (Branco and Dey 2001; Azzalini and Capitanio 2003; Gupta 2003), skew-Cauchy distribution, skew-slash distribution (Wang and Genton 2006), and the skew-slash-t distribution (Punathumparambath 2012), for example. In this chapter, we present a unified family of asymmetric distributions that offers extreme flexibility by combining both skewness with heavy tails. This family contains, as a special case, the multivariate skew-normal distribution defined by Azzalini and Dalla-Valle (1996), the multivariate skew-slash distribution defined by Wang and Genton (2006), the multivariate skew-t distribution defined by Azzalini and Capitanio (2003), and all the distributions studied by Lange and Sinsheimer (1993) in a symmetric context.

3.2 SMN Distributions

The symmetric family of SMN distributions has attracted much attention in the last few years, mainly because they include distributions such as the Student-t, the slash, the power exponential, and the contaminated normal distributions. All these distributions have heavier tails than the normal. We say that a p-dimensional vector $\mathbf{Y}$ has an SMN distribution (Andrews and Mallows 1974; Lange and Sinsheimer 1993) with location parameter $\boldsymbol{\mu}$ and a positive definite scale matrix $\boldsymbol{\Sigma}$, if its pdf assumes the form

$$f(\mathbf{y}) = \int_0^\infty \phi_p(y|\boldsymbol{\mu}, u^{-1}\boldsymbol{\Sigma})dH(u; \boldsymbol{\nu}), \tag{3.5}$$

where $H(u; \boldsymbol{\nu})$ is a cdf of a unidimensional positive random variable U indexed by a parameter vector $\boldsymbol{\nu}$. The random variable U is called the *scale factor* and $H(u; \boldsymbol{\nu})$ is the *mixture distribution*. For a random vector with a pdf as in (3.5), we use the notation $\mathbf{Y} \sim \text{SMN}_p(\boldsymbol{\mu}, \boldsymbol{\Sigma}; H)$. When $\boldsymbol{\mu} = \mathbf{0}$ and $\boldsymbol{\Sigma} = \mathbf{I}_p$, we get a standard SMN distribution and use the notation $\mathbf{Y} \sim \text{SMN}_p(H)$. A stochastic representation is given by

$$\mathbf{Y} = \boldsymbol{\mu} + U^{-1/2}\mathbf{Z}, \tag{3.6}$$

where $\mathbf{Z} \sim \text{N}_p(\mathbf{0}, \boldsymbol{\Sigma})$ and U is a positive random variable, independent of $\mathbf{Z}$, with cdf H . Examples of SMN distributions are described subsequently, as well as the distributional properties of the squared Mahalanobis distance $d = (\mathbf{y}-\boldsymbol{\mu})^\top\boldsymbol{\Sigma}^{-1}(\mathbf{y}-\boldsymbol{\mu})$, which is extremely useful in testing the goodness of fit and detecting outliers.

3.2.1 Examples of SMN Distributions

- *The Student-t distribution with* $\nu > 0$ *degrees of freedom,* $\mathbf{Y} \sim \text{t}_p(\boldsymbol{\mu}, \boldsymbol{\Sigma}, \nu)$. The use of the t-distribution as an alternative to the normal distribution has frequently been suggested in the literature; Little (1988) and Lange et al. (1989), for example, used the Student-t distribution for robust modeling. The density of $\mathbf{Y}$ is given by

$$f(\mathbf{y}) = \frac{\Gamma\left(\frac{p+\nu}{2}\right)}{\Gamma\left(\frac{\nu}{2}\right)\pi^{p/2}}\nu^{-p/2}|\boldsymbol{\Sigma}|^{-1/2}\left(1 + \frac{d}{\nu}\right)^{-\left(\frac{p+\nu}{2}\right)}. \tag{3.7}$$

  In this case, we have that $U \sim \text{Gamma}(\nu/2, \nu/2)$, where $H(u; \nu)$ has density

$$h(u; \nu) = \frac{(\nu/2)^{\nu/2}u^{\nu/2-1}}{\Gamma(\nu/2)}\exp\left(-\frac{\nu}{2}u\right),$$

  with finite reciprocal moments $\text{E}[U^{-m}] = \dfrac{(\nu/2)^m\Gamma(\nu/2 - m)}{\Gamma(\nu/2)}$, for $m < \nu/2$. From Lange and Sinsheimer (1993), it also follows that $d \sim pF(p, \nu)$, where $F(p, \nu)$ denotes the F distribution with parameters p and ν.
- *The slash distribution,* $\mathbf{Y} \sim \text{SL}_p(\boldsymbol{\mu}, \boldsymbol{\Sigma}, \nu)$, *with shape parameter* $\nu > 0$ (Rogers and Tukey 1972).

This distribution has heavier tails than those of the normal distribution and it includes the normal case when $\nu \uparrow \infty$. Its pdf is given by

$$f(\mathbf{y}) = \nu \int_0^1 u^{\nu-1} \phi_p(\mathbf{y}|\boldsymbol{\mu}, u^{-1}\boldsymbol{\Sigma}) du.$$

Here U has a Beta distribution with parameters ν and 1, with density

$$h(u; \nu) = \nu u^{\nu-1} \mathbb{I}_{(0,1)}(u), \tag{3.8}$$

where $\mathbb{I}_A(\cdot)$ is the indicator function of the set A, with reciprocal moments $\mathrm{E}[U^{-m}] = \dfrac{\nu}{\nu - m}$, for $m < \nu$. The distribution of d is given by

$$\Pr(d \leq r) = \Pr\left(\chi_p^2 \leq r\right) - \frac{2^\nu \Gamma(p/2 + \nu)}{r^\nu \Gamma(p/2)} Pr\left(\chi_{p+2\nu}^2 \leq r\right),$$

where χ_p^2 denotes a random variable with chi-square distribution with p degrees of freedom.

- *The contaminated normal distribution,* $\mathbf{Y} \sim \mathrm{CN}_p(\boldsymbol{\mu}, \boldsymbol{\Sigma}, \nu, \gamma)$, $0 < \nu < 1$, $0 < \gamma < 1$ (Aitkin and Wilson 1980). This distribution may also be applied for modeling symmetric data with outlying observations. The parameter ν represents the percentage of outliers, while γ is a scale factor. Its pdf is given by

$$f(\mathbf{y}) = \nu \phi_p\left(\mathbf{y}|\boldsymbol{\mu}, \frac{\boldsymbol{\Sigma}}{\gamma}\right) + (1 - \nu)\phi_p(\mathbf{y}|\boldsymbol{\mu}, \boldsymbol{\Sigma}).$$

In this case U is a discrete random variable with probability function

$$h(u; \boldsymbol{\nu}) = \nu \mathbb{I}_{\{\gamma\}}(u) + (1 - \nu)\mathbb{I}_{\{1\}}(1), \quad \boldsymbol{\nu} = (\nu, \gamma)^\top. \tag{3.9}$$

We have $\mathrm{E}[U^{-m}] = \nu/\gamma^m + 1 - \nu$, and

$$\Pr(d \leq r) = \nu \Pr\left(\chi_p^2 \leq \gamma r\right) + (1 - \nu)\Pr\left(\chi_p^2 \leq r\right).$$

3.3 Multivariate SMSN Distributions and Main Results

In this section, we define the multivariate SMSN distributions and study some of its important properties, viz., moments, kurtosis, linear transformations, and marginal and conditional distributions.

Definition 3.1 A p-dimensional random vector $\mathbf{Y}$ follows an SMSN distribution with location parameter $\boldsymbol{\mu}$ positive definite scale matrix and shape parameter $\boldsymbol{\lambda}$ if its pdf is given by

$$f(\mathbf{y}) = 2\int_0^\infty \phi_p(\mathbf{y}|\boldsymbol{\mu}, u^{-1}\boldsymbol{\Sigma})\Phi\big(u^{1/2}\boldsymbol{\lambda}^\top\boldsymbol{\Sigma}^{-1/2}(\mathbf{y}-\boldsymbol{\mu})\big)dH(u;\boldsymbol{\nu}), \tag{3.10}$$

where $H(u;\boldsymbol{\nu})$ is a cdf of a unidimensional positive random variable U indexed by a parameter vector $\boldsymbol{\nu}$.

If $\mathbf{Y}$ has a pdf as in (3.10), we use the notation $\mathbf{Y} \sim \text{SMSN}_p(\boldsymbol{\mu}, \boldsymbol{\Sigma}, \boldsymbol{\lambda}; H)$. When $\boldsymbol{\mu} = \mathbf{0}$ and $\boldsymbol{\Sigma} = \mathbf{I}_p$ we get a standard SMSN distribution and denote it by $\text{SMSN}_p(\boldsymbol{\lambda}; H)$. When $\boldsymbol{\lambda} = \mathbf{0}$ we get back the SMN class of distributions defined in (3.5). If we suppose that $\boldsymbol{\nu}_\infty$ is such that $\boldsymbol{\nu} \uparrow \boldsymbol{\nu}_\infty$, and $H(u;\boldsymbol{\nu})$ converges weakly to the distribution function $H_\infty(u) = H(u;\boldsymbol{\nu}_\infty)$ of the unit point mass at 1, then the density function in (3.10) converges to the density function of a random vector having a skew-normal distribution. The proof of this result is similar to that of Lange and Sinsheimer (1993) for the SMN case.

For an SMSN random vector, the stochastic representation given below can be used to simulate pseudorealizations of $\mathbf{Y}$ and also to study many of its properties.

Proposition 3.1 *Let* $\mathbf{Y} \sim SMSN_p(\boldsymbol{\mu}, \boldsymbol{\Sigma}, \boldsymbol{\lambda}; H)$. *Then*

$$\mathbf{Y} \stackrel{d}{=} \boldsymbol{\mu} + U^{-1/2}\mathbf{Z}, \tag{3.11}$$

where $\mathbf{Z} \sim SN_p(\mathbf{0}, \boldsymbol{\Sigma}, \boldsymbol{\lambda})$ *and* U *is a positive random variable with cdf* H *independent of* $\mathbf{Z}$.

Proof The proof follows from the fact that $\mathbf{Y}|U = u \sim \text{SN}_p(\boldsymbol{\mu}, u^{-1}\boldsymbol{\Sigma}, \boldsymbol{\lambda})$. □

Notice that the stochastic representation given in (3.6) for the SMN case is a special case of (3.11) when $\boldsymbol{\lambda} = \mathbf{0}$. Hence, we have extended the family of SMN distributions for the skewed case. Besides, from (3.3) it follows that (3.11) can be written as

$$\mathbf{Y} \stackrel{d}{=} \boldsymbol{\mu} + \frac{1}{U^{1/2}}\boldsymbol{\Sigma}^{1/2}\left\{\boldsymbol{\delta}|X_0| + \left(\mathbf{I}_p - \boldsymbol{\delta}\boldsymbol{\delta}^T\right)^{1/2}\mathbf{X}_1\right\}, \tag{3.12}$$

where $\boldsymbol{\delta} = \boldsymbol{\lambda}/\sqrt{1+\boldsymbol{\lambda}^\top\boldsymbol{\lambda}}$, and U, $X_0 \sim N(0,1)$ and $\mathbf{X}_1 \sim \text{N}_p(\mathbf{0}, \mathbf{I}_p)$ are all independent. The marginal stochastic representation given in (3.12) is very important since it allows to implement the EM algorithm for a wide variety of linear models similar to those presented in Lachos et al. (2010).

In the next proposition, we derive a general expression for the moment generating function (mgf) of an SMSN random vector.

Proposition 3.2 *Let* $\mathbf{Y} \sim SMSN_p(\boldsymbol{\mu}, \boldsymbol{\Sigma}, \boldsymbol{\lambda}; H)$. *Then*

$$M_{\mathbf{Y}}(\mathbf{s}) = E[e^{\mathbf{s}^\top\mathbf{Y}}] = \int_0^\infty 2e^{\mathbf{s}^\top\boldsymbol{\mu} + \frac{1}{2}u^{-1}\mathbf{s}^\top\boldsymbol{\Sigma}\mathbf{s}}\Phi\big(u^{-1/2}\boldsymbol{\delta}^\top\boldsymbol{\Sigma}^{1/2}\mathbf{s}\big)dH(u), \quad \mathbf{s} \in \mathbb{R}^p.$$

Proof From Proposition 3.1, we have that $\mathbf{Y}|U = u \sim \mathrm{SN}_p(\boldsymbol{\mu}, u^{-1}\boldsymbol{\Sigma}, \boldsymbol{\lambda})$. From known properties of conditional expectation, it follows that $M_{\mathbf{y}}(\mathbf{s}) = \mathrm{E}_U[\mathrm{E}[e^{\mathbf{s}^\top \mathbf{Y}}|U]]$, where E_U denotes expectation with respect to the distribution of U. From (3.4), we have that $\mathrm{E}[e^{\mathbf{s}^\top \mathbf{Y}}|U = u] = 2e^{u^{-1}\mathbf{s}^\top \boldsymbol{\mu} + \frac{1}{2}\mathbf{s}^\top \boldsymbol{\Sigma}\mathbf{s}}\Phi(u^{-1/2}\boldsymbol{\delta}^\top \boldsymbol{\Sigma}^{1/2}\mathbf{s})$. □

In the next proposition we show that the SMSN family is closed under affine transformations. In particular, marginal distributions are still SMSN.

Proposition 3.3 *Let* $\mathbf{Y} \sim SMSN_p(\boldsymbol{\mu}, \boldsymbol{\Sigma}, \boldsymbol{\lambda}; H)$. *Then for any fixed vector* $\mathbf{b} \in \mathbb{R}^m$ *and matrix* $\mathbf{A} : m \times p$ *of full row rank matrix,*

$$\mathbf{b} + \mathbf{A}\mathbf{Y} \sim SMSN_p\big(\mathbf{b} + \mathbf{A}\boldsymbol{\mu}, \mathbf{A}\boldsymbol{\Sigma}\mathbf{A}^\top, \boldsymbol{\lambda}^*; H\big),$$

where $\boldsymbol{\lambda}^* = \boldsymbol{\delta}^*/\big(1 - \boldsymbol{\delta}^{*\top}\boldsymbol{\delta}^*\big)^{1/2}$, *with* $\boldsymbol{\delta}^* = \big(\mathbf{A}\boldsymbol{\Sigma}\mathbf{A}^\top\big)^{-1/2}\mathbf{A}\boldsymbol{\Sigma}^{1/2}\boldsymbol{\delta}$.

Proof Let $\boldsymbol{\Omega} = \mathbf{A}\boldsymbol{\Sigma}\mathbf{A}^\top$. From Proposition 3.2, we have that

$$\begin{aligned}\mathrm{M}_{\mathbf{b}+\mathbf{A}\mathbf{Y}}(\mathbf{s}) &= e^{\mathbf{s}^\top \mathbf{b}}\mathrm{M}_{\mathbf{Y}}\big(\mathbf{A}^\top \mathbf{s}\big)\\ &= \int_0^\infty 2e^{\mathbf{s}^\top(\mathbf{b}+\mathbf{A}\boldsymbol{\mu}) + \frac{1}{2}u^{-1}\mathbf{s}^\top \boldsymbol{\Omega}\mathbf{s}}\Phi\big(u^{-1/2}\boldsymbol{\delta}^\top \boldsymbol{\Sigma}^{1/2}\mathbf{A}^\top \boldsymbol{\Omega}^{-1/2}\boldsymbol{\Omega}^{1/2}\mathbf{s}\big)dH(u),\end{aligned}$$

proving the assertion. □

By using Proposition 3.3, with $\mathbf{A} = [\mathbf{I}_{p_1}, \mathbf{0}_{p_2}]$, $p_1 + p_2 = p$, we obtain the marginal distribution of an SMSN random vector.

Corollary 3.1 *Let* $\mathbf{Y} \sim SMSN_p(\boldsymbol{\mu}, \boldsymbol{\Sigma}, \boldsymbol{\lambda}; H)$ $\mathbf{Y}$ *be partitioned as* $\mathbf{Y}^\top = (\mathbf{Y}_1^\top, \mathbf{Y}_2^\top)^\top$ *of dimensions* p_1 *and* p_2 $(p_1 + p_2 = p)$, *respectively; let*

$$\boldsymbol{\Sigma} = \begin{pmatrix}\boldsymbol{\Sigma}_{11} & \boldsymbol{\Sigma}_{12}\\ \boldsymbol{\Sigma}_{21} & \boldsymbol{\Sigma}_{22}\end{pmatrix}, \quad \boldsymbol{\mu} = \big(\boldsymbol{\mu}_1^\top, \boldsymbol{\mu}_2^\top\big)^\top$$

be the corresponding partitions of $\boldsymbol{\Sigma}$ *and* $\boldsymbol{\mu}$. *Then, the marginal distribution of* $\mathbf{Y}_1$ *is* $SMSN_{p_1}(\boldsymbol{\mu}_1, \boldsymbol{\Sigma}_{11}, \boldsymbol{\Sigma}_{11}^{1/2}\widetilde{\boldsymbol{\upsilon}}; H)$, *where*

$$\widetilde{\boldsymbol{\upsilon}} = \frac{\boldsymbol{\upsilon}_1 + \boldsymbol{\Sigma}_{11}^{-1}\boldsymbol{\Sigma}_{12}\boldsymbol{\upsilon}_2}{\sqrt{1 + \boldsymbol{\upsilon}_2^\top \boldsymbol{\Sigma}_{22.1}\boldsymbol{\upsilon}_2}}.$$

with $\boldsymbol{\Sigma}_{22.1} = \boldsymbol{\Sigma}_{22} - \boldsymbol{\Sigma}_{21}\boldsymbol{\Sigma}_{11}^{-1}\boldsymbol{\Sigma}_{12}$, $\boldsymbol{\upsilon} = \boldsymbol{\Sigma}^{-1/2}\boldsymbol{\lambda} = \big(\boldsymbol{\upsilon}_1^\top, \boldsymbol{\upsilon}_2^\top\big)^\top$.

Lemma 3.1 *Let* $\mathbf{Y} \in \mathbb{R}^p$ *a random vector with the following pdf*

$$f(\mathbf{y}|u) = k^{-1}(u)\phi_p(\mathbf{y}|\boldsymbol{\mu}, u^{-1}\boldsymbol{\Sigma})\Phi\big(u^{1/2}A + u^{1/2}\mathbf{B}^\top \mathbf{y}\big),$$

where u is a positive constant, $A \in \mathbb{R}$, $\mathbf{B}$ any fixed p-dimensional vector and $k(u) = \Phi\left(u^{1/2}\frac{A+\mathbf{B}^\top\boldsymbol{\mu}}{\sqrt{1+\mathbf{B}^\top\boldsymbol{\Sigma}\mathbf{B}}}\right)$ is a standardized constant. Then,

$$E[\mathbf{Y}|u] = \boldsymbol{\mu} + u^{-1/2}\frac{\boldsymbol{\Sigma}\mathbf{B}}{\sqrt{1+\mathbf{B}^\top\boldsymbol{\Sigma}\mathbf{B}}}W_\Phi\left(u^{1/2}\frac{A+\mathbf{B}^\top\boldsymbol{\mu}}{\sqrt{1+\mathbf{B}^\top\boldsymbol{\Sigma}\mathbf{B}}}\right),$$

where $W_\Phi(x) = \phi(x)/\Phi(x)$.

Proof First note, by using Lemma 2 from Arellano-Valle et al. (2005), that

$$\begin{aligned}
\mathrm{E}[\mathbf{Y}|u] &= k^{-1}(u)\int_{\mathbb{R}}\int_0^\infty \mathbf{y}\phi_1\big(t|u^{1/2}A + u^{1/2}\mathbf{B}^\top\mathbf{y}, 1\big)\phi\big(\mathbf{y}|\boldsymbol{\mu}, u^{-1}\boldsymbol{\Sigma}\big)dtd\mathbf{y} \\
&= k^{-1}(u)\int_0^\infty \phi_1\big(t|u^{1/2}A + u^{1/2}\mathbf{B}^\top\boldsymbol{\mu}, 1+\mathbf{B}^\top\boldsymbol{\Sigma}\mathbf{B}\big)E_{\mathbf{Y}|t}[\mathbf{Y}]dt,
\end{aligned}$$

where $\mathbf{Y}|t \sim \mathrm{N}_p(\boldsymbol{\mu} - \boldsymbol{\Lambda}\mathbf{B}(A+\mathbf{B}^\top\boldsymbol{\mu}) + u^{-1/2}\boldsymbol{\Lambda}\mathbf{B}t, u^{-1}\boldsymbol{\Lambda})$, with $\boldsymbol{\Lambda} = (\boldsymbol{\Sigma}^{-1} + \mathbf{B}\mathbf{B}^\top)^{-1}$, and the proof follows by using known properties of the truncated normal distribution. □

Proposition 3.4 *Under the notation of Corollary 3.1, if $\mathbf{Y} \sim SMSN_p(\boldsymbol{\mu}, \boldsymbol{\Sigma}, \boldsymbol{\lambda}; H)$ then the distribution of $\mathbf{Y}_2$ conditionally on $\mathbf{Y}_1 = \mathbf{y}_1$ and $U = u$ has density given by*

$$f(\mathbf{y}_2|\mathbf{y}_1, u) = \phi_{p_2}\big(\mathbf{y}_2|\boldsymbol{\mu}_{2.1}, u^{-1}\boldsymbol{\Sigma}_{22.1}\big)\frac{\Phi\big(u^{1/2}\boldsymbol{\upsilon}^\top(\mathbf{y}-\boldsymbol{\mu})\big)}{\Phi\big(u^{1/2}\widetilde{\boldsymbol{\upsilon}}^\top(\mathbf{y}_1-\boldsymbol{\mu}_1)\big)}, \tag{3.13}$$

with $\boldsymbol{\mu}_{2.1} = \boldsymbol{\mu}_2 + \boldsymbol{\Sigma}_{21}\boldsymbol{\Sigma}_{11}^{-1}(\mathbf{y}_1 - \boldsymbol{\mu}_1)$. Furthermore,

$$\mathrm{E}[\mathbf{Y}_2|\mathbf{y}_1, u] = \boldsymbol{\mu}_{2.1} + u^{-1/2}\frac{\phi\big(u^{1/2}\widetilde{\boldsymbol{\upsilon}}^\top(\mathbf{y}_1-\boldsymbol{\mu}_1)\big)}{\Phi\big(u^{1/2}\widetilde{\boldsymbol{\upsilon}}^\top(\mathbf{y}_1-\boldsymbol{\mu}_1)\big)}\frac{\boldsymbol{\Sigma}_{22.1}\boldsymbol{\upsilon}_2}{\sqrt{1+\boldsymbol{\upsilon}_2^\top\boldsymbol{\Sigma}_{22.1}\boldsymbol{\upsilon}_2}}. \tag{3.14}$$

Proof In fact, the density of $f(\mathbf{y}_2|\mathbf{y}_1, u) = f(\mathbf{y}|u)/f(\mathbf{y}_1|u)$, and (3.13) follows by noting that $\mathbf{Y}|U = u \sim \mathrm{SN}_p(\boldsymbol{\mu}, u^{-1}\boldsymbol{\Sigma}, \boldsymbol{\lambda})$ and $\mathbf{Y}_1|U = u \sim \mathrm{SN}(\boldsymbol{\mu}_1, u^{-1}\boldsymbol{\Sigma}_{11}, \boldsymbol{\Sigma}_{11}^{1/2}\widetilde{\boldsymbol{\upsilon}})$. Result (3.14) follows from Lemma 3.1, with $A = \boldsymbol{\upsilon}_1^\top(\mathbf{y}_1 - \boldsymbol{\mu}_1) - \boldsymbol{\upsilon}_2^\top\boldsymbol{\mu}_2$, $\mathbf{B} = \boldsymbol{\upsilon}_2$, $\boldsymbol{\mu} = \boldsymbol{\mu}_{2.1}$ and $\boldsymbol{\Sigma} = \boldsymbol{\Sigma}_{22.1}$, which concludes the proof. □

Note that given u, when $\boldsymbol{\Sigma}_{21} = \mathbf{0}$ and $\boldsymbol{\lambda}_2 = \mathbf{0}$, is possible to obtain independence for the components $\mathbf{Y}_1$ and $\mathbf{Y}_2$ of an SMSN random vector $\mathbf{Y}$. The following corollary is a by-product of Proposition 3.4, since $E[\mathbf{Y}_2|\mathbf{y}_1] = E_U[E[\mathbf{Y}_2|\mathbf{y}_1, U]|\mathbf{y}_1]$.

Proposition 3.5 *Consider the notation of Corollary 3.1. If* $\mathbf{Y} \sim SMSN_p(\boldsymbol{\mu}, \boldsymbol{\Sigma}, \boldsymbol{\lambda}; H)$*, then the first moment of* $\mathbf{Y}_2$ *conditionally on* $\mathbf{Y}_1 = \mathbf{y}_1$ *is given by*

$$E[\mathbf{Y}_2|\mathbf{y}_1] = \boldsymbol{\mu}_{2.1} + \frac{\boldsymbol{\Sigma}_{22.1}\boldsymbol{\upsilon}_2}{\sqrt{1+\boldsymbol{\upsilon}_2^\top \boldsymbol{\Sigma}_{22.1}\boldsymbol{\upsilon}_2}} E\left[U^{-1/2}\frac{\phi_1(U^{1/2}\widetilde{\boldsymbol{\upsilon}}^\top(\mathbf{y}_1-\boldsymbol{\mu}_1))}{\Phi_1(U^{1/2}\widetilde{\boldsymbol{\upsilon}}^\top(\mathbf{y}_1-\boldsymbol{\mu}_1))}|\mathbf{y}_1\right],$$

with $\boldsymbol{\mu}_{2.1} = \boldsymbol{\mu}_2 + \boldsymbol{\Sigma}_{21}\boldsymbol{\Sigma}_{11}^{-1}(\mathbf{y}_1 - \boldsymbol{\mu}_1)$.

In Sect. 3.3.1, we give additional results for some elements of this family of distributions based on Proposition 3.5. The next result can be useful in applications to linear models. For instance, when the linear model depends on a vector of unobservable random effects and a vector of random errors (linear mixed model), in which the random effects is assumed to have an SMSN distribution and the errors are assumed to have an SMN distribution (see, for instance, Lachos et al. 2010).

Proposition 3.6 *Let* $\mathbf{X} \sim SMSN_m(\boldsymbol{\mu}_1, \boldsymbol{\Sigma}_1, \boldsymbol{\lambda}, H)$ *and* $\mathbf{Y} \sim SMN_p(\boldsymbol{\mu}_2, \boldsymbol{\Sigma}_2, H)$*, where for a positive random variable* U *with cdf* H*, we can write* $\mathbf{X} \stackrel{d}{=} \boldsymbol{\mu}_1 + U^{-1/2}\mathbf{Z}$ *and* $\mathbf{Y} \stackrel{d}{=} \boldsymbol{\mu}_2 + U^{-1/2}\mathbf{W}$*, with* $\mathbf{Z} \sim SN_m(\mathbf{0}, \boldsymbol{\Sigma}_1, \boldsymbol{\lambda})$ *independent of* $\mathbf{W} \sim N_p(\mathbf{0}, \boldsymbol{\Sigma}_2)$*, then for any matrix* $\mathbf{A}$ *of dimension* $p \times m$*,*

$$\mathbf{AX} + \mathbf{Y} \sim SMSN_m(\mathbf{A}\boldsymbol{\mu}_1 + \boldsymbol{\mu}_2, \mathbf{A}\boldsymbol{\Sigma}_1\mathbf{A}^\top + \boldsymbol{\Sigma}_2, \boldsymbol{\lambda}_*; H),$$

where $\boldsymbol{\lambda}_* = \boldsymbol{\delta}_*/\sqrt{1-\boldsymbol{\delta}_*^\top\boldsymbol{\delta}_*}$*, with* $\boldsymbol{\delta}_* = (\mathbf{A}\boldsymbol{\Sigma}_1\mathbf{A}^\top + \boldsymbol{\Sigma}_2)^{-1/2}\mathbf{A}\boldsymbol{\Sigma}_1^{1/2}\boldsymbol{\delta}$.

Proof The proof is based on the result of Proposition 3.2. Note first that given U; $\mathbf{X}$ and $\mathbf{Y}$ are independent, so that letting $\mathbf{V} = \mathbf{AX} + \mathbf{Y}$, we have that

$$\begin{aligned}
M_{\mathbf{V}}(\mathbf{s}) &= E_U\left(E\left[e^{\mathbf{s}^\top\mathbf{AX}}|U\right]E\left[e^{\mathbf{s}^\top\mathbf{Y}}|U\right]\right) \\
&= \int_0^\infty 2\mathrm{e}^{\mathbf{s}^\top\mathbf{A}\boldsymbol{\mu}_1 + \frac{1}{2u}\mathbf{s}^\top\mathbf{A}\boldsymbol{\Sigma}_1\mathbf{A}^\top\mathbf{s}}\,\Phi\left(\frac{\boldsymbol{\delta}^\top\boldsymbol{\Sigma}_1^{1/2}\mathbf{A}^\top\mathbf{s}}{\sqrt{u}}\right)e^{\mathbf{s}^\top\boldsymbol{\mu}_2 + \frac{1}{2u}\mathbf{s}^\top\boldsymbol{\Sigma}_2\mathbf{s}}\,dH(u) \\
&= \int_0^\infty 2\mathrm{e}^{\mathbf{s}^\top(\mathbf{A}\boldsymbol{\mu}_1+\boldsymbol{\mu}_2) + \frac{1}{2u}\mathbf{s}^\top(\mathbf{A}\boldsymbol{\Sigma}_1\mathbf{A}^\top + \boldsymbol{\Sigma}_2)\mathbf{s}}\,\Phi\left(\frac{\boldsymbol{\delta}^\top\boldsymbol{\Sigma}_1^{1/2}\mathbf{A}^\top\mathbf{s}}{\sqrt{u}}\right)dH(u) \\
&= \int_0^\infty 2\mathbf{e}^{\mathbf{t}^\top(\mathbf{A}\boldsymbol{\mu}_1+\boldsymbol{\mu}_2) + \frac{1}{2u}\mathbf{s}^\top(\mathbf{A}\boldsymbol{\Sigma}_1\mathbf{A}^\top + \boldsymbol{\Sigma}_2)\mathbf{s}}\,\Phi\left(\frac{\boldsymbol{\delta}_*^\top\boldsymbol{\Psi}^{1/2}\mathbf{s}}{\sqrt{u}}\right)dH(u),
\end{aligned}$$

where $\boldsymbol{\Psi} = \mathbf{A}\boldsymbol{\Sigma}_1\mathbf{A}^\top + \boldsymbol{\Sigma}_2$ and where $\boldsymbol{\delta}_* = \boldsymbol{\Psi}^{-1/2}\mathbf{A}\boldsymbol{\Sigma}_1^{1/2}\boldsymbol{\delta}$, and the proof follows from Proposition 3.2. □

In the following proposition we derive the mean vector and the covariance matrix of an SMSN random vector. Moreover, we present the multidimensional kurtosis coefficient for a random vector SMSN, which represents an extension of the kurtosis coefficient proposed by Azzalini and Capitanio (1999). Before we give the following Lemma:

Lemma 3.2 *Let* $\mathbf{Y} \sim SN_p(\boldsymbol{\lambda})$. *Then for any fixed p-dimensional vector* $\mathbf{b}$ *and* $p \times p$ *matrix* $\mathbf{A}$,

$$E\big[\mathbf{Y}^\top \mathbf{A}\mathbf{Y}\mathbf{b}^\top \mathbf{Y}\big] = -\sqrt{\frac{2}{\pi}}\big[(\boldsymbol{\delta}^\top \mathbf{A}\boldsymbol{\delta} + tr(\mathbf{A}))\mathbf{b}^\top \boldsymbol{\delta} + 2\boldsymbol{\delta}^\top \mathbf{A}\mathbf{b}\big],$$

where $\boldsymbol{\delta}$ *is as in (3.12).*

Proof The proof follows by using the stochastic representation of $\mathbf{Y}$ given in (3.3) and of the moments $E[|X_0|]$ and $E[|X_0|^3]$, where $X_0 \sim N(0, 1)$. □

Proposition 3.7 *Suppose that* $\mathbf{Y} \sim SMSN_p(\boldsymbol{\mu}, \boldsymbol{\Sigma}, \boldsymbol{\lambda}; H)$. *Then,*

a) If $E[U^{-1/2}] < \infty$, *then* $E[\mathbf{Y}] = \boldsymbol{\mu} + \sqrt{\frac{2}{\pi}} E[U^{-1/2}]\boldsymbol{\Sigma}^{1/2}\boldsymbol{\delta}$;
b) If $E[U^{-1}] < \infty$, *then* $Var[\mathbf{Y}] = \boldsymbol{\Sigma}_y = E[U^{-1}]\boldsymbol{\Sigma} - \frac{2}{\pi}E^2[U^{-1/2}]\boldsymbol{\Sigma}^{1/2}\boldsymbol{\delta}\boldsymbol{\delta}^\top\boldsymbol{\Sigma}^{1/2}$;
c) If $E[U^{-2}] < \infty$, *then the multidimensional kurtosis coefficient is*

$$\gamma_2(\mathbf{Y}) = \frac{E\big[U^{-2}\big]}{E^2\big[U^{-1}\big]}a_{1y} - 4\frac{E\big[U^{-3/2}\big]}{E^2\big[U^{-1}\big]}a_{2y} + a_{3y} - p(p+2),$$

where $a_{1y} = p(p+2) + 2(p+2)\boldsymbol{\mu}_y^\top \boldsymbol{\Sigma}_y^{-1}\boldsymbol{\mu}_y + 3(\boldsymbol{\mu}_y^\top \boldsymbol{\Sigma}_y^{-1}\boldsymbol{\mu}_y)^2$, $a_{2y} = \left(p + \frac{2}{E[U^{-1/2}]}\right)\boldsymbol{\mu}_y^\top \boldsymbol{\Sigma}_y^{-1}\boldsymbol{\mu}_y + \left(1 + \frac{2}{E[U^{-1/2}]} - \frac{\pi}{2}\frac{E[U^{-1}]}{E^2[U^{-1/2}]}\right)(\boldsymbol{\mu}_y^\top \boldsymbol{\Sigma}_y^{-1}\boldsymbol{\mu}_y)^2$, *and* $a_{3y} = 2(p+2)\boldsymbol{\mu}_y^\top \boldsymbol{\Sigma}_y^{-1}\boldsymbol{\mu}_y + 3(\boldsymbol{\mu}_y^\top \boldsymbol{\Sigma}_y^{-1}\boldsymbol{\mu}_y)^2$, *with* $\boldsymbol{\mu}_y = E[\mathbf{Y} - \boldsymbol{\mu}] = \sqrt{\frac{2}{\pi}}E[U^{-1/2}]\boldsymbol{\Sigma}^{1/2}\boldsymbol{\delta}$.

Proof The proof of a) and b) follows from Proposition 3.1. To obtain the expression in c), we use the definition of the multivariate kurtosis introduced by Mardia (1970). Without loss of generality, we consider that $\boldsymbol{\mu} = \mathbf{0}$, so that $\boldsymbol{\mu}_y = E[\mathbf{Y}] = \sqrt{\frac{2}{\pi}}E[U^{-1/2}]\boldsymbol{\Sigma}^{1/2}\boldsymbol{\delta}$. Note first that the kurtosis is defined by $\gamma_2(\mathbf{Y}) = E[\{(\mathbf{Y} - \boldsymbol{\mu}_y)^\top \boldsymbol{\Sigma}_y^{-1}(\mathbf{Y} - \boldsymbol{\mu}_y)\}^2]$. Now, by using the stochastic representation of $\mathbf{Y}$ given in (3.6), we have that

$$(\mathbf{Y} - \boldsymbol{\mu}_y)^\top \boldsymbol{\Sigma}_y^{-1}(\mathbf{Y} - \boldsymbol{\mu}_y) \stackrel{d}{=} U^{-1}\mathbf{Z}^\top \boldsymbol{\Sigma}_y^{-1}\mathbf{Z} - 2U^{-1/2}\mathbf{Z}^\top \boldsymbol{\Sigma}_y^{-1}\boldsymbol{\mu}_y + \boldsymbol{\mu}_y^\top \boldsymbol{\Sigma}_y^{-1}\boldsymbol{\mu}_y,$$

where $\mathbf{Z} \sim SN_p(\mathbf{0}, \boldsymbol{\Sigma}, \boldsymbol{\lambda})$. According to definition of $\gamma_2(\mathbf{Y})$ and after some algebraic manipulations, the proof follows by using of the first two moments of a quadratic form (see Genton et al. 2001) along with Lemma 3.2. □

Notice that under the skew-normal distribution, i.e., when $U = 1$, the multidimensional kurtosis coefficient reduces to $\gamma_2(\mathbf{Y}) = 2(\pi - 3)(\boldsymbol{\mu}_y^\top \boldsymbol{\Sigma}_y^{-1} \boldsymbol{\mu}_y)^2$, which is the kurtosis coefficient for a skew-normal random vector (see, for instance, Azzalini and Capitanio 1999).

Proposition 3.8 *If* $\mathbf{Y} \sim SMSN_p(\boldsymbol{\mu}, \boldsymbol{\Sigma}, \boldsymbol{\lambda}; H)$*, then for any even function* g*, the distribution of* $g(\mathbf{Y} - \boldsymbol{\mu})$ *does not depend on* $\boldsymbol{\lambda}$ *and has the same distribution that* $g(\mathbf{X} - \boldsymbol{\mu})$*, where* $\mathbf{X} \sim SMN_p(\boldsymbol{\mu}, \boldsymbol{\Sigma}; H)$*. In a particular case, if* $\mathbf{A}$ *is a* $p \times p$ *symmetric matrix, then* $(\mathbf{Y} - \boldsymbol{\mu})^\top \mathbf{A}(\mathbf{Y} - \boldsymbol{\mu})$ *and* $(\mathbf{X} - \boldsymbol{\mu})^\top \mathbf{A}(\mathbf{X} - \boldsymbol{\mu})$ *are identically distributed.*

Proof The proof follows by using Proposition 3.2 and a similar procedure to found in Wang et al. (2004). □

As a by-product of Proposition 3.8, we have the following: interesting result

Corollary 3.2 *Let* $\mathbf{Y} \sim SMSN_p(\boldsymbol{\mu}, \boldsymbol{\Sigma}, \boldsymbol{\lambda}; H)$*. Then the quadratic form*

$$d = (\mathbf{Y} - \boldsymbol{\mu})^\top \boldsymbol{\Sigma}^{-1} (\mathbf{Y} - \boldsymbol{\mu})$$

has the same distribution as $d^* = (\mathbf{X} - \boldsymbol{\mu})^\top \boldsymbol{\Sigma}^{-1} (\mathbf{X} - \boldsymbol{\mu})$*, where* $\mathbf{X} \sim SMN_p(\boldsymbol{\mu}, \boldsymbol{\Sigma}; H)$*.*

The result of Corollary 3.2 is interesting because it allows us to check models in practice. On the other hand, Corollary 3.2 together with the result found in Lange and Sinsheimer (1993) allows us to obtain the mth moment of d_λ.

Corollary 3.3 *Let* $\mathbf{Y} \sim SMSN_p(\boldsymbol{\mu}, \boldsymbol{\Sigma}, \boldsymbol{\lambda}; H)$*. Then for any* $m > 0$

$$E\big[d_\lambda^m\big] = \frac{2^m \Gamma(m + p/2)}{\Gamma(p/2)} E[U^{-m}].$$

3.3.1 Examples of SMSN Distributions

Some examples of SMSN distributions include

- *The skew-t distribution, with* ν *degrees of freedom*, $\mathrm{ST}_p(\boldsymbol{\mu}, \boldsymbol{\Sigma}, \boldsymbol{\lambda}, \nu)$. Considering $U \sim \mathrm{Gamma}(\nu/2, \nu/2)$, similar procedures found in Gupta (2003, Section 2) lead to the following density function:

$$f(\mathbf{y}) = 2\mathrm{t}_p(\mathbf{y}|\boldsymbol{\mu}, \boldsymbol{\Sigma}, \nu)\mathrm{T}_1\left(\frac{\sqrt{\nu + p}\boldsymbol{\lambda}^\top \boldsymbol{\Sigma}^{-1/2}(\mathbf{y} - \boldsymbol{\mu})}{\sqrt{d + \nu}}|0, 1, \nu + p\right), \quad \mathbf{y} \in \mathbb{R}^p, \tag{3.15}$$

  where $\mathrm{t}_p(\cdot|\boldsymbol{\mu}, \boldsymbol{\Sigma}, \nu)$ and $\mathrm{T}_p(\cdot|\boldsymbol{\mu}, \boldsymbol{\Sigma}, \nu)$ denote, respectively, the pdf and cdf of the Student-t distribution, $t_p(\boldsymbol{\mu}, \boldsymbol{\Sigma}, \nu)$, defined in (3.7). A particular case of the skew-t distribution is the skew-Cauchy distribution, when $\nu = 1$. Also, when

$\nu \uparrow \infty$, we get the skew-normal distribution as the limiting case. See Gupta (2003) for further details. In this case, from Proposition 3.7, the mean and covariance matrix of $\mathbf{Y} \sim \mathrm{ST}_p(\boldsymbol{\mu}, \boldsymbol{\Sigma}, \boldsymbol{\lambda}, \nu)$ are given by

$$\mathrm{E}[\mathbf{Y}] = \boldsymbol{\mu} + \sqrt{\frac{\nu}{\pi}} \frac{\Gamma(\frac{\nu-1}{2})}{\Gamma(\frac{\nu}{2})} \boldsymbol{\Sigma}^{1/2}\boldsymbol{\delta}, \quad \nu > 1 \text{ and}$$

$$\mathrm{Var}[\mathbf{Y}] = \frac{\nu}{\nu-2}\boldsymbol{\Sigma} - \frac{\nu}{\pi}\left(\frac{\Gamma(\frac{\nu-1}{2})}{\Gamma(\frac{\nu}{2})}\right)^2 \boldsymbol{\Sigma}^{1/2}\boldsymbol{\delta}\boldsymbol{\delta}^\top\boldsymbol{\Sigma}^{1/2}, \quad \nu > 2.$$

In what follows, we give an important result which will be used in the implementation of the EM algorithm for mixture models and to find closed form expressions of the first conditional moment given in Proposition 3.5.

Proposition 3.9 *If* $\mathbf{Y} \sim \mathrm{ST}_p(\boldsymbol{\mu}, \boldsymbol{\Sigma}, \boldsymbol{\lambda}, \nu)$, *then*

$$E[U^r|\mathbf{y}] = \frac{2^{r+1}\nu^{\nu/2}\Gamma\left(\frac{p+\nu+2r}{2}\right)(d+\nu)^{-\frac{p+\nu+2r}{2}}}{f(\mathbf{y})\Gamma(\nu/2)\sqrt{\pi^p}|\boldsymbol{\Sigma}|^{1/2}} T_1\left(\sqrt{\frac{p+\nu+2r}{d+\nu}}A|0, 1, p+\nu+2r\right)$$

and

$$E[U^r W_{\Phi_1}(U^{1/2}A)|\mathbf{y}] = \frac{2^{r+1/2}\nu^{\nu/2}\Gamma\left(\frac{p+\nu+2r}{2}\right)\left(d+\nu+A^2\right)^{-\frac{p+\nu+2r}{2}}}{f(\mathbf{y})\Gamma(\nu/2)\sqrt{\pi}^{p+1}|\boldsymbol{\Sigma}|^{1/2}}.$$

where $A = \boldsymbol{\lambda}^\top\boldsymbol{\Sigma}^{-1/2}(\mathbf{y}-\boldsymbol{\mu})$.

Proof The proof follows from Lemma 1 given Azzalini and Capitanio (2003), since $f(u|\mathbf{y}) = f(\mathbf{y}, u)/f(\mathbf{y})$ and

$$\mathrm{E}[U^r|\mathbf{y}] = \frac{2}{f(\mathbf{y})}\int_0^\infty u^r\phi_p(\mathbf{y}|\boldsymbol{\mu}, u^{-1}\boldsymbol{\Sigma})\Phi_1(u^{1/2}A)G_u(\nu/2, \nu/2)du,$$

and

$$\mathrm{E}[U^r W_{\Phi_1}(U^{1/2}A)|\mathbf{y}] = \frac{2}{f(\mathbf{y})}\int_0^\infty u^r\phi_p(\mathbf{y}|\boldsymbol{\mu}, u^{-1}\boldsymbol{\Sigma})\phi_1(u^{1/2}A)G_u(\nu/2, \nu/2)du,$$

where $G_u(\nu/2, \nu/2)$ denotes the pdf of the Gamma$(\frac{\nu}{2}, \frac{\nu}{2})$ distribution. □

For a skew-t random vector $\mathbf{Y}$, partitioned as $\mathbf{Y}^\top = (\mathbf{Y}_1^\top, \mathbf{Y}_2^\top)^\top$, we have from Corollary 1 that $\mathbf{Y}_1 \sim \mathrm{ST}_{p_1}(\boldsymbol{\mu}_1, \boldsymbol{\Sigma}_{11}, \boldsymbol{\Sigma}_{11}^{1/2}\widetilde{\boldsymbol{\upsilon}}, \nu)$. Thus, from Proposition 3.5 we have the following result:

Corollary 3.4 *Under the notation of Proposition 3.5, if* $\mathbf{Y} \sim \mathrm{ST}_p(\boldsymbol{\mu}, \boldsymbol{\Sigma}, \boldsymbol{\lambda}, \nu)$*, then*

$$E[\mathbf{Y}_2|\mathbf{y}_1] = \boldsymbol{\mu}_{2.1} + \frac{\boldsymbol{\Sigma}_{22.1}\boldsymbol{\upsilon}_2}{\sqrt{1+\boldsymbol{\upsilon}_2^\top \boldsymbol{\Sigma}_{22.1}\boldsymbol{\upsilon}_2}}$$
$$\times \frac{1}{f(\mathbf{y}_1)} \frac{\nu^{\nu/2}\Gamma\left(\frac{\nu+p_1-1}{2}\right)}{\Gamma(\nu/2)\sqrt{\pi}^{(p_1+1)}|\boldsymbol{\Sigma}_{11}|^{1/2}}$$
$$\left(\nu + d_{y_1} + (\widetilde{\boldsymbol{\upsilon}}^\top(\mathbf{y}_1 - \boldsymbol{\mu}_1))^2\right)^{-\frac{\nu+p_1-1}{2}}$$

where $d_{y_1} = (\mathbf{y}_1 - \boldsymbol{\mu}_1)^\top \boldsymbol{\Sigma}_{11}^{-1}(\mathbf{y}_1 - \boldsymbol{\mu}_1)$.

- *The skew-slash distribution, with the shape parameter* $\nu > 0$, $\mathrm{SSL}_p(\boldsymbol{\mu}, \boldsymbol{\Sigma}, \boldsymbol{\lambda}, \nu)$. With $h(u; \nu)$ as in (3.8), from the Proposition 3.1, can be easily seen that

$$f(\mathbf{y}) = 2\nu \int_0^1 u^{\nu-1}\phi_p\left(\mathbf{y}|\boldsymbol{\mu}, \frac{\boldsymbol{\Sigma}}{u}\right)\Phi_1(u^{1/2}\boldsymbol{\lambda}^\top\boldsymbol{\Sigma}^{-1/2}(\mathbf{y}-\boldsymbol{\mu})), \quad \mathbf{y} \in \mathbb{R}^p, \tag{3.16}$$

The skew-slash distribution reduces to the skew-normal distribution when $\nu \uparrow \infty$. See Wang and Genton (2006) for further details. In this case, from Proposition 3.7

$$E[\mathbf{Y}] = \boldsymbol{\mu} + \sqrt{\frac{2}{\pi}}\frac{2\nu}{2\nu-1}\boldsymbol{\Sigma}^{1/2}\boldsymbol{\delta}, \quad \nu > 1/2, \quad \text{and}$$

$$Var[\mathbf{Y}] = \frac{\nu}{\nu-1}\boldsymbol{\Sigma} - \frac{2}{\pi}\left(\frac{2\nu}{2\nu-1}\right)^2 \boldsymbol{\Sigma}^{1/2}\boldsymbol{\delta}\boldsymbol{\delta}^\top\boldsymbol{\Sigma}^{1/2}, \quad \nu > 1.$$

As in the skew-t case we have the following results:

Proposition 3.10 *If* $\mathbf{Y} \sim SSL_p(\boldsymbol{\mu}, \boldsymbol{\Sigma}, \boldsymbol{\lambda}, \nu)$*, then*

$$E[U^r|\mathbf{y}] = \frac{2^{\nu+r+1}\nu\Gamma\left(\frac{p+2\nu+2r}{2}\right)P_1\left(\frac{p+2\nu+2r}{2}, \frac{d}{2}\right)d^{-\frac{p+2\nu+2r}{2}}}{f(\mathbf{y})\sqrt{\pi^p}|\boldsymbol{\Sigma}|^{1/2}} E[\Phi(S^{1/2}A)],$$

where $S_i \sim Gamma\left(\frac{p+2\nu+2r}{2}, \frac{d}{2}\right)\mathbb{I}_{(0,1)}$ *and*

$$E[U^r W_{\Phi_1}(U^{1/2}A)|\mathbf{y}]$$
$$= \frac{2^{\nu+r+1/2}\nu\Gamma\left(\frac{2\nu+p+2r}{2}\right)}{f(\mathbf{y})\sqrt{\pi}^{p+1}|\boldsymbol{\Sigma}|^{1/2}}(d+A^2)^{-\frac{2\nu+p+2r}{2}} P_1\left(\frac{2\nu+p+2r}{2}, \frac{d+A^2}{2}\right)$$

where $P_x(a,b)$ denotes the cdf of the Gamma(a,b) distribution evaluated at x.

Corollary 3.5 *Under the notation of Proposition 3.5, if $\mathbf{Y} \sim SSL_p(\boldsymbol{\mu}, \boldsymbol{\Sigma}, \boldsymbol{\lambda}, \nu)$, then*

$$E[\mathbf{Y}_2|\mathbf{y}_1] = \boldsymbol{\mu}_{2.1} + \frac{\boldsymbol{\Sigma}_{22.1}\boldsymbol{\upsilon}_2}{\sqrt{1+\boldsymbol{\upsilon}_2^\top\boldsymbol{\Sigma}_{22.1}\boldsymbol{\upsilon}_2}}$$
$$\times \frac{2^\nu\nu}{f(\mathbf{y}_1)} \frac{\Gamma\frac{(p_1+2\nu-1)}{2}\left(d_{y1}+(\widetilde{\boldsymbol{\upsilon}}^\top(\mathbf{y}_1-\boldsymbol{\mu}_1))^2\right)^{-\frac{p_1+2\nu-1}{2}}}{\sqrt{\pi}^{(p_1+1)}|\boldsymbol{\Sigma}_{11}|^{1/2}}$$
$$\times P_1\left(\frac{p_1+2\nu-1}{2}, \frac{d_{y_1}+(\widetilde{\boldsymbol{\upsilon}}^\top(\mathbf{y}_1-\boldsymbol{\mu}_1))^2}{2}\right),$$

where $d_{y_1} = (\mathbf{y}_1-\boldsymbol{\mu}_1)^\top\boldsymbol{\Sigma}_{11}^{-1}(\mathbf{y}_1-\boldsymbol{\mu}_1)$.

- *The skew-contaminated normal distribution, $SCN_p(\boldsymbol{\mu}, \boldsymbol{\Sigma}, \boldsymbol{\lambda}, \nu, \gamma)$, $0<\nu<1$,* $0<\gamma<1$. Taking $h(u;\boldsymbol{\nu})$ as in (3.9), it follows straightforwardly that

$$f(\mathbf{y}) = 2\left\{\nu\phi_p\left(\mathbf{y}|\boldsymbol{\mu}, \frac{\boldsymbol{\Sigma}}{\gamma}\right)\Phi_1(\gamma^{1/2}\boldsymbol{\lambda}^\top\boldsymbol{\Sigma}^{-1/2}(\mathbf{y}-\boldsymbol{\mu}))\right.$$
$$\left.+(1-\nu)\phi_p(\mathbf{y}|\boldsymbol{\mu},\boldsymbol{\Sigma})\Phi_1(\boldsymbol{\lambda}^\top\boldsymbol{\Sigma}^{-1/2}(\mathbf{y}-\boldsymbol{\mu}))\right\}, \quad (3.17)$$

in this case, the skew-contaminated normal distribution reduces to the skew-normal distribution when $\gamma = 1$. Hence, the mean vector and the covariance matrix are given, respectively, by

$$E[\mathbf{Y}] = \boldsymbol{\mu} + \sqrt{\frac{2}{\pi}}\left(\frac{\nu}{\gamma^{1/2}}+1-\nu\right)\boldsymbol{\Sigma}^{1/2}\boldsymbol{\delta}, \text{ and}$$

$$Var[\mathbf{Y}] = \left(\frac{\nu}{\gamma}+1-\nu\right)\boldsymbol{\Sigma} - \frac{2}{\pi}\left(\frac{\nu}{\gamma^{1/2}}+1-\nu\right)^2\boldsymbol{\Sigma}^{1/2}\boldsymbol{\delta}\boldsymbol{\delta}^\top\boldsymbol{\Sigma}^{1/2}.$$

From (3.17) it follows the following results

Proposition 3.11 *If* $\mathbf{Y} \sim SCN_p(\boldsymbol{\mu}, \boldsymbol{\Sigma}, \boldsymbol{\lambda}, \nu, \gamma)$*, then*

$$E[U^r|\mathbf{y}] = \frac{2}{f(\mathbf{y})}\left[\nu\gamma^r\phi_p(\mathbf{y}|\boldsymbol{\mu}, \gamma^{-1}\boldsymbol{\Sigma})\Phi_1(\gamma^{1/2}A) + (1-\nu)\phi_p(\mathbf{y}|\boldsymbol{\mu}, \boldsymbol{\Sigma})\Phi_1(A)\right]$$

and

$$E[U^r W_{\Phi_1}(U^{1/2}A)|\mathbf{y}] = \frac{2}{f(\mathbf{y})}\Big[\nu\gamma^r\phi_p(\mathbf{y}|\boldsymbol{\mu}, \gamma^{-1}\boldsymbol{\Sigma})\phi_1(\gamma^{1/2}A)$$
$$+(1-\nu)\phi_p(\mathbf{y}|\boldsymbol{\mu}, \boldsymbol{\Sigma})\phi_1(A)\Big].$$

Corollary 3.6 *Under the notation of Proposition 3.5, if* $\mathbf{Y} \sim SCN_p(\boldsymbol{\mu}, \boldsymbol{\Sigma}, \boldsymbol{\lambda}, \nu, \gamma)$*, then*

$$E[\mathbf{Y}_2|\mathbf{y}_1] = \boldsymbol{\mu}_{2.1} + \frac{2\boldsymbol{\Sigma}_{22.1}\boldsymbol{\upsilon}_2}{f(\mathbf{y}_1)\sqrt{1+\boldsymbol{\upsilon}_2^\top\boldsymbol{\Sigma}_{22.1}\boldsymbol{\upsilon}_2}}$$
$$\times\Big[\nu\gamma^{-1/2}\phi_{p_1}(\mathbf{y}_1|\boldsymbol{\mu}_1, \gamma^{-1}\boldsymbol{\Sigma}_{11})\phi_1(\gamma^{1/2}\widetilde{\boldsymbol{\upsilon}}^\top(\mathbf{y}_1-\boldsymbol{\mu}_1))$$
$$+(1-\nu)\phi_{p_1}(\mathbf{y}_1|\boldsymbol{\mu}_1, \boldsymbol{\Sigma}_{11})\phi_1(\widetilde{\boldsymbol{\upsilon}}^\top(\mathbf{y}_1-\boldsymbol{\mu}_1))\Big],$$

where $d_{y_1} = (\mathbf{y}_1-\boldsymbol{\mu}_1)^\top\boldsymbol{\Sigma}_{11}^{-1}(\mathbf{y}_1-\boldsymbol{\mu}_1)$.

In Fig. 3.1, we depict the density of the standard distribution $\mathrm{SN}_1(3)$ together with the standard densities of the distributions $\mathrm{ST}_1(3, 2)$, $\mathrm{SSL}_1(3, 1)$, and $\mathrm{SNC}_1(3, 0.5, 0.5)$. They are rescaled so that they have the same value at the origin. Note that the four densities are positively skewed, and that the skew-slash and the skew-t distributions have much heavier tails than the skew-normal distribution. Figure 3.2 depicts some contours of the densities associated with the standard bivariate skew-normal distribution $SN_2(\boldsymbol{\lambda})$, the standard bivariate skew-t distribution $\mathrm{ST}_2(\boldsymbol{\lambda}, 2)$, the standard bivariate skew-slash distribution $\mathrm{SSL}_2(\boldsymbol{\lambda}, 1)$, and the standard bivariate skew-contaminated normal distribution $\mathrm{SCN}_2(\boldsymbol{\lambda}, 0.5, 0.5)$, with $\boldsymbol{\lambda} = (2, 1)^\top$ for all the distributions. Note that these contours are not elliptical and they can be strongly asymmetric depending on the choice of the parameters.

3.3.2 A Simulation Study

To illustrate the usefulness of the SMSN distribution, we perform a small simulation to study the behavior of two location estimators, the sample mean and the sample median, under four different standard univariate settings. In particular, we consider a standard skew-normal $\mathrm{SN}_1(3)$, a skew-t $\mathrm{ST}_1(3, 2)$, a skew-slash $\mathrm{SSL}_1(3, 1)$,

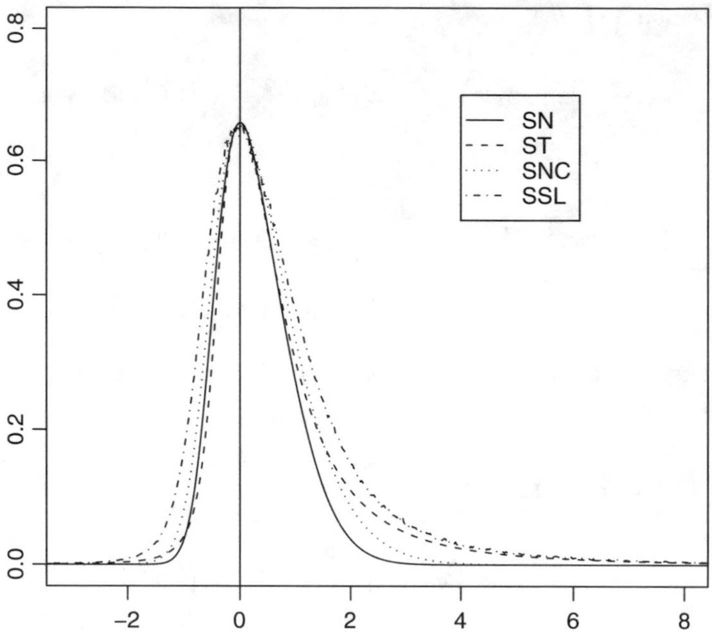

Fig. 3.1 Densities curves of the univariate skew-normal, skew-t, skew-slash, and skew-contaminated normal distributions

and a skew-contaminated normal $\mathrm{SCN}_1(3, 0.9, 0.1)$. The mean of all asymmetric distributions is adjusted to zero, so that all four distributions are comparable. Thus, this setting represents four distributions with the same mean, but with different tail behaviors and skewness. Note that the skew-slash and skew-t will have infinite variance when $\nu = 1$ and 2, respectively. We simulate 500 samples of size $n = 100$ from each of these four distributions. For each sample, we compute the sample mean and the sample median and report the boxplot for each distribution in Fig. 3.3. In the left panel, we observe that all boxplots of the estimated means are centered around zero but have larger variability for the heavy-tailed distributions (skew-t and skew-slash). In the right panel, we see that the boxplots of the estimated medians has a slightly larger variability for the skew-normal and skew-contaminated normal and has a much smaller variability for skew-t and skew-slash distributions. This indicates that the median is a robust estimator of location at asymmetric light tailed distributions. On the other hand, the median estimator becomes biased as soon as unexpected skewness and heavy-tailed arise in the underlying distribution.

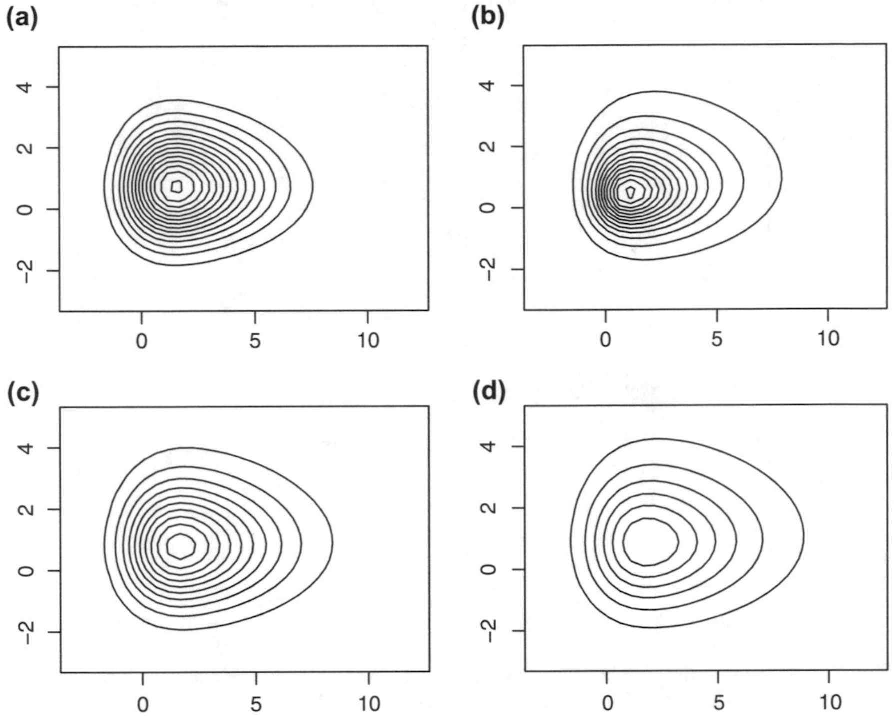

Fig. 3.2 Contour plot of some elements of the standard bivariate SMSN family. (**a**) $SN_2(\boldsymbol{\lambda})$, (**b**) $ST_2(\boldsymbol{\lambda}, 2)$, (**c**) $SCN_2(\boldsymbol{\lambda}, 0.5, 0.5)$, (**d**) $SSL_2(\boldsymbol{\lambda}, 1)$, where $\boldsymbol{\lambda} = (2, 1)^\top$

3.4 Maximum Likelihood Estimation

This section presents an EM algorithm for performing maximum likelihood estimation for multivariate SMSN responses. EM algorithms for particular cases of the skew-normal and skew-t distributions were considered in Lin (2009, 2010) (see also Lachos et al. 2007), respectively.

Suppose that we have observations on n independent subjects, $\mathbf{Y}_1, \ldots, \mathbf{Y}_n$, where $\mathbf{Y}_i \sim SMSN_p(\boldsymbol{\mu}, \boldsymbol{\Sigma}, \boldsymbol{\lambda}; H)$, $i = 1, \ldots, n$. The parameter vector is defined to be $\boldsymbol{\theta} = (\boldsymbol{\mu}^\top, \boldsymbol{\alpha}^\top, \boldsymbol{\lambda}^\top)^\top$, where $\boldsymbol{\alpha}$ denotes a minimal set of parameters such that $\boldsymbol{\Sigma}(\boldsymbol{\alpha})$ is well defined (e.g., the upper triangular elements of $\boldsymbol{\Sigma}$ in the unstructured case).

In what follows, we illustrate the implementation of likelihood inference for the multivariate SMSN via the EM algorithm. Notice that, by using (3.12), the set-up defined above can be written as

$$\mathbf{Y}_i | T_i = t_i, U_i = u_i, \overset{\text{ind}}{\sim} N_p\big(\boldsymbol{\mu} + t_i \boldsymbol{\Sigma}^{1/2}\boldsymbol{\delta}, u_i^{-1}\boldsymbol{\Sigma}^{1/2}(\mathbf{I}_p - \boldsymbol{\delta}\boldsymbol{\delta}^\top)\boldsymbol{\Sigma}^{1/2}\big), \quad (3.18)$$

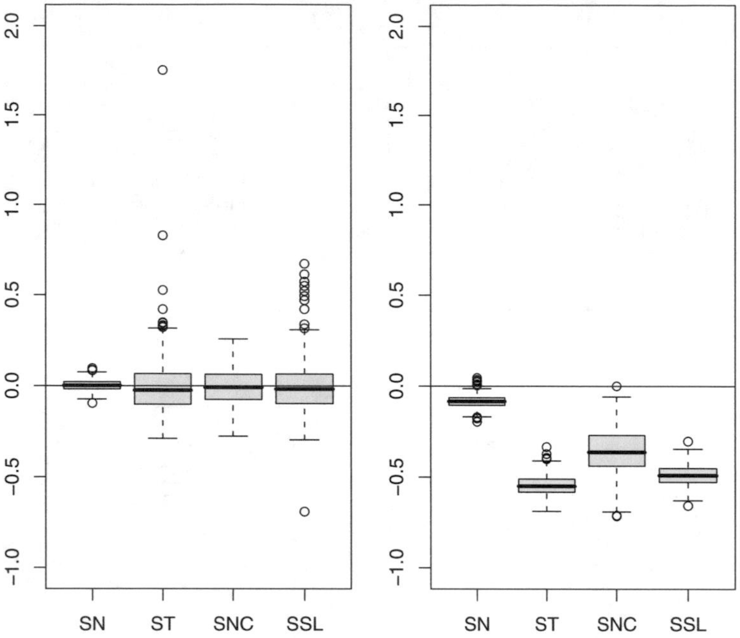

Fig. 3.3 Boxplots of the sample mean (left panel) and sample median (right panel) on 500 samples of size $n = 100$ from the four standardized distributions: $\text{SN}_1(3)$; $\text{ST}_1(3, 2)$; $\text{SSL}_1(3, 1)$, and $\text{SNC}_1(3, 0.9, 0.1)$. The respective means are adjusted to zero

$$T_i|U_i = u_i \overset{\text{iid}}{\sim} HN\big(0, u_i^{-1}\big) \tag{3.19}$$

$$U_i \overset{\text{ind}}{\sim} h(u_i; \boldsymbol{\nu}), \tag{3.20}$$

$i = 1, \ldots, n$, all independent, where $HN(0, 1)$ denotes the univariate standard half-normal distribution. We assume that the parameter vector $\boldsymbol{\nu}$ is known. In applications the optimum value of $\boldsymbol{\nu}$ can be determined using the profile likelihood and the Schwarz information criterion (see Lange and Sinsheimer 1993).

Let $\mathbf{y} = (\mathbf{y}_1^\top, \ldots, \mathbf{y}_n^\top)^\top$ $\mathbf{u} = (u_1, \ldots, u_n)^\top$ and $\mathbf{t} = (t_1, \ldots, t_n)^\top$. Then, under the hierarchical representation (3.18)–(3.20), with $\boldsymbol{\Delta} = \boldsymbol{\Sigma}^{1/2}\boldsymbol{\delta}$ and $\boldsymbol{\Gamma} = \boldsymbol{\Sigma} - \boldsymbol{\Delta}\boldsymbol{\Delta}^\top$, it follows that the complete log-likelihood function associated with $\mathbf{y}_c = (\mathbf{y}^\top, \mathbf{u}^\top, \mathbf{t}^\top)^\top$ is

$$\begin{aligned} &\ell_c(\boldsymbol{\theta}|\mathbf{y}_c) \\ &= c - \frac{n}{2}\log|\boldsymbol{\Gamma}| - \frac{1}{2}\sum_{i=1}^{n} u_i(\mathbf{y}_i - \boldsymbol{\mu} - \boldsymbol{\Delta}t_i)^\top\boldsymbol{\Gamma}^{-1}(\mathbf{y}_i - \boldsymbol{\mu} - \boldsymbol{\Delta}t_i) \end{aligned} \tag{3.21}$$

where c is a constant that is independent of the parameter vector $\boldsymbol{\theta}$. Letting $\widehat{u}_i = \mathrm{E}[U_i|\boldsymbol{\theta} = \widehat{\boldsymbol{\theta}}, \mathbf{y}_i]$, $\widehat{ut}_i = \mathrm{E}[U_iT_i|\boldsymbol{\theta} = \widehat{\boldsymbol{\theta}}, \mathbf{y}_i]$, $\widehat{ut_i^2} = \mathrm{E}[U_iT_i^2|\boldsymbol{\theta} = \widehat{\boldsymbol{\theta}}, \mathbf{y}_i]$ and using known properties of conditional expectation we obtain

$$\widehat{ut}_i = \widehat{u}_i\widehat{\mu}_{Ti} + \widehat{M}_{T_i}\widehat{\eta}_i \tag{3.22}$$

$$\widehat{ut^2}_i = \widehat{u}_i\widehat{\mu}^2_{T_i} + \widehat{M}^2_{T_i} + \widehat{M}_{T_i}\widehat{\mu}_{T_i}\widehat{\eta}_i, \tag{3.23}$$

where $\widehat{\eta}_i = E\left[U_i^{1/2}W_{\Phi_1}\left(\frac{U_i^{1/2}\widehat{\mu}_{T_i}}{\widehat{M}_{T_i}}\right)|\widehat{\boldsymbol{\theta}}, \mathbf{y}_i\right]$, $W_{\Phi_1}(x) = \phi_1(x)/\Phi_1(x)$, $\widehat{M}^2_T = 1/(1 + \widehat{\boldsymbol{\Delta}}^\top\widehat{\boldsymbol{\Gamma}}^{-1}\widehat{\boldsymbol{\Delta}})$ and $\widehat{\mu}_{T_i} = \widehat{M}^2_{T_i}\widehat{\boldsymbol{\Delta}}^\top\widehat{\boldsymbol{\Gamma}}^{-1}(\mathbf{y}_i - \boldsymbol{\mu})$, $i = 1, \ldots, n$.

Since $\frac{\mu_{T_i}}{M_{T_i}} = \boldsymbol{\lambda}^\top\boldsymbol{\Sigma}^{-1/2}(\mathbf{y}_i - \boldsymbol{\mu})$, the conditional expectations given in (3.22) and (3.23), specifically $\widehat{u}_i$ and $\widehat{\eta}_i$, can be easily derived from the results given in Sect. 3.3.1. Thus, at least for the skew-t and skew-contaminated normal distributions of the SMSN class we have closed form expressions for the quantities $\widehat{u}_i$ and $\widehat{\eta}_i$. For the skew-slash case, Monte Carlo integration may be employed, which yields the so-called MC-EM algorithm.

It follows, after some simple algebra and using (3.22)–(3.23), that the conditional expectation of the complete log-likelihood function has the form

$$Q(\boldsymbol{\theta}|\widehat{\boldsymbol{\theta}}) = \mathrm{E}\big[\ell_c(\boldsymbol{\theta}|\mathbf{y}_c)|\mathbf{y}, \widehat{\boldsymbol{\theta}}\big] = c - \frac{n}{2}\log|\boldsymbol{\Gamma}| - \frac{1}{2}\sum_{i=1}^n \widehat{u}_i(\mathbf{y}_i - \boldsymbol{\mu})^\top\boldsymbol{\Gamma}^{-1}(\mathbf{y}_i - \boldsymbol{\mu})$$
$$+ \sum_{i=1}^n \widehat{ut}_i(\mathbf{y}_i - \boldsymbol{\mu})^\top\boldsymbol{\Gamma}^{-1}\boldsymbol{\Delta} - \frac{1}{2}\sum_{i=1}^n \widehat{ut^2}_i\boldsymbol{\Delta}^\top\boldsymbol{\Gamma}^{-1}\boldsymbol{\Delta}.$$

Then, we have the following EM-type algorithm:

E-Step Given $\boldsymbol{\theta} = \widehat{\boldsymbol{\theta}}$, compute $\widehat{ut^2}_i$, $\widehat{ut}_i$ and $\widehat{u}_i$, for $i = 1, \ldots, n$, using (3.22) and (3.23).

M-Step Update $\widehat{\boldsymbol{\theta}}$ by maximizing $Q(\boldsymbol{\theta}|\widehat{\boldsymbol{\theta}})$ over $\boldsymbol{\theta}$, which leads to the following closed form expressions

$$\widehat{\boldsymbol{\mu}} = \sum_{i=1}^n \left(\widehat{u}_i\mathbf{y}_i - \widehat{ut}_i\boldsymbol{\Delta}\right)/\left(\sum_{i=1}^n \widehat{u}_i\right), \tag{3.24}$$

$$\widehat{\boldsymbol{\Gamma}} = \frac{1}{n}\sum_{i=1}^n \left[\widehat{u}_i(\mathbf{y}_i - \boldsymbol{\mu})(\mathbf{y}_i - \boldsymbol{\mu})^\top - 2\widehat{ut}_i\boldsymbol{\Delta}(\mathbf{y}_i - \boldsymbol{\mu})^\top + \widehat{ut^2}_i\boldsymbol{\Delta}\boldsymbol{\Delta}^\top\right],$$

$$\widehat{\boldsymbol{\Delta}} = \frac{\sum_{i=1}^n \widehat{ut}_i(\mathbf{y}_i - \boldsymbol{\mu})}{\sum_{i=1}^n \widehat{ut^2}_i}.$$

The skewness parameter vector and the unstructured scale matrix can be estimated by noting that $\widehat{\boldsymbol{\Sigma}} = \widehat{\boldsymbol{\Gamma}} + \widehat{\boldsymbol{\Delta}}\widehat{\boldsymbol{\Delta}}^T$ and $\widehat{\boldsymbol{\lambda}} = \widehat{\boldsymbol{\Sigma}}^{-1/2}\widehat{\boldsymbol{\Delta}}/(1-\widehat{\boldsymbol{\Delta}}^\top\widehat{\boldsymbol{\Sigma}}^{-1}\widehat{\boldsymbol{\Delta}})^{1/2}$. It is clear that when $\boldsymbol{\lambda} = \mathbf{0}$ (or $\boldsymbol{\Delta} = \mathbf{0}$) the M-step equations reduce to the equations obtained assuming an SMN distribution. Note also that this algorithm clearly generalized the results found in Lachos et al. (2007, Section 2) by taking $U_i = 1, i = 1, \ldots, n$. Useful starting values required to implement this algorithm are those obtained under the normality assumption, with the starting values for the skewness parameter vector set equal to $\mathbf{0}$. However, in order to ensure that the true ML estimate is identified, we recommend running the EM algorithm using a range of different starting values. The log-likelihood function for $\boldsymbol{\theta} = (\boldsymbol{\mu}^\top, \boldsymbol{\alpha}^\top, \boldsymbol{\lambda}^\top)^\top$, given the observed sample $\mathbf{y} = (\mathbf{y}_1^\top, \ldots, \mathbf{y}_n^\top)^\top$ is of the form

$$\ell(\boldsymbol{\theta}) = \sum_{i=1}^{n} \ell_i(\boldsymbol{\theta}), \tag{3.25}$$

where $\ell_i(\boldsymbol{\theta}) = \log 2 - \frac{p}{2} log 2\pi - \frac{1}{2}\log|\boldsymbol{\Sigma}| + \log K_i$, with

$$K_i = K_i(\boldsymbol{\theta}) = \int_0^\infty u_i^{p/2} \exp\left\{-\frac{1}{2}u_i d_i\right\} \Phi_1\left(u_i^{1/2} A_i\right) dH(u_i),$$

where $d_i = (\mathbf{y}_i - \boldsymbol{\mu})^\top \boldsymbol{\Sigma}^{-1}(\mathbf{y}_i - \boldsymbol{\mu})$ and $A_i = \boldsymbol{\lambda}^\top \boldsymbol{\Sigma}^{-1}(\mathbf{y}_i - \boldsymbol{\mu})$.

3.5 The Observed Information Matrix

In this section we develop the observed information matrix in a general form. Suppose that we have observations on n independent individuals, $\mathbf{Y}_1, \ldots, \mathbf{Y}_n$, where $\mathbf{Y}_i \sim \text{SMSN}_p(\boldsymbol{\mu}, \boldsymbol{\Sigma}, \boldsymbol{\lambda}; H)$, $i = 1, \ldots, n$. Then, the log-likelihood function for $\boldsymbol{\theta} = (\boldsymbol{\mu}^\top, \boldsymbol{\alpha}^\top, \boldsymbol{\lambda}^\top)^\top \in \mathbb{R}^q$, given the observed sample $\mathbf{y} = (\mathbf{y}_1^\top, \ldots, \mathbf{y}_n^\top)^\top$, is of the form

$$\ell(\boldsymbol{\theta}) = \sum_{i=1}^{n} \ell_i(\boldsymbol{\theta}), \tag{3.26}$$

where $\ell_i(\boldsymbol{\theta}) = \log 2 - \frac{n_i}{2}\log 2\pi - \frac{1}{2}\log|\boldsymbol{\Sigma}| + \log K_i$, with

$$K_i = K_i(\boldsymbol{\theta}) = \int_0^\infty u_i^{n_i/2} \exp\left\{-\frac{1}{2}u_i d_i\right\} \Phi_1(u_i^{1/2} A_i) dH(u_i),$$

and $d_i = (\mathbf{y}_i - \boldsymbol{\mu})^\top \boldsymbol{\Sigma}^{-1}(\mathbf{y}_i - \boldsymbol{\mu})$, $A_i = \boldsymbol{\lambda}_i^\top \boldsymbol{\Sigma}^{-1}(\mathbf{y}_i - \boldsymbol{\mu})$. Using the notation

$$I_i^{\Phi}(w) = \int_0^{\infty} u_i^w \exp\left\{-\frac{1}{2}u_i d_i\right\} \Phi_1(u_i^{1/2}A_i) dH(u_i),$$

$$I_i^{\phi}(w) = \int_0^{\infty} u_i^w \exp\left\{-\frac{1}{2}u_i d_i\right\} \phi_1(u_i^{1/2}A_i|0,1) dH(u_i),$$

so that $K_i(\boldsymbol{\theta})$ can be expressed as $K_i(\boldsymbol{\theta}) = I_i^{\Phi}(\frac{n_i}{2})$, $i = 1, \ldots, n$, it follows that the matrix of second derivatives with respect to $\boldsymbol{\theta}$ is given by

$$\mathbf{L} = \sum_{i=1}^{n} \frac{\partial^2 \ell_i(\boldsymbol{\theta})}{\partial\boldsymbol{\theta}\partial\boldsymbol{\theta}^\top} = -\frac{1}{2}\sum_{i=1}^{n} \frac{\partial^2 \log|\boldsymbol{\Sigma}_i|}{\partial\boldsymbol{\theta}\partial\boldsymbol{\theta}^\top} - \sum_{i=1}^{n} \frac{1}{K_i^2}\frac{\partial K_i}{\partial\boldsymbol{\theta}}\frac{\partial K_i}{\partial\boldsymbol{\theta}^\top} + \sum_{i=1}^{n} \frac{1}{K_i}\frac{\partial^2 K_i}{\partial\boldsymbol{\theta}\partial\boldsymbol{\theta}^\top}, \tag{3.27}$$

where

$$\frac{\partial K_i}{\partial\boldsymbol{\theta}} = I_i^{\phi}\left(\frac{n_i+1}{2}\right)\frac{\partial A_i}{\partial\boldsymbol{\theta}} - \frac{1}{2}I_i^{\Phi}\left(\frac{n_i+2}{2}\right)\frac{\partial d_i}{\partial\boldsymbol{\theta}}$$

and

$$\begin{aligned}\frac{\partial^2 K_i}{\partial\boldsymbol{\theta}\partial\boldsymbol{\theta}^\top} &= \frac{1}{4}I_i^{\Phi}\left(\frac{n_i+4}{2}\right)\frac{\partial d_i}{\partial\boldsymbol{\theta}}\frac{\partial d_i}{\partial\boldsymbol{\theta}^\top} - \frac{1}{2}I_i^{\Phi}\left(\frac{n_i+2}{2}\right)\frac{\partial^2 d_i}{\partial\boldsymbol{\theta}\partial\boldsymbol{\theta}^\top} \\ &\quad -\frac{1}{2}I_i^{\phi}\left(\frac{n_i+3}{2}\right)\left(\frac{\partial A_i}{\partial\boldsymbol{\theta}}\frac{\partial d_i}{\partial\boldsymbol{\theta}^\top} + \frac{\partial d_i}{\partial\boldsymbol{\theta}}\frac{\partial A_i}{\partial\boldsymbol{\theta}^\top}\right) - I_i^{\phi}\left(\frac{n_i+3}{2}\right)A_i\frac{\partial A_i}{\partial\boldsymbol{\theta}}\frac{\partial A_i}{\partial\boldsymbol{\theta}^\top} \\ &\quad +I_i^{\Phi}\left(\frac{n_i+1}{2}\right)\frac{\partial^2 A_i}{\partial\boldsymbol{\theta}\partial\boldsymbol{\theta}^\top}.\end{aligned} \tag{3.28}$$

From Propositions 3.8–3.10 we have that, for each distribution considered in this work, the integrals above can be written as

- *Skew-t.*

$$I_i^{\Phi}(w) = \frac{2^w \nu^{\nu/2}\Gamma(w+\nu/2)}{\Gamma(\nu/2)(\nu+d_i)^{\nu/2+w}} T_1\left(\frac{A_i}{(d_i+\nu)^{1/2}}\sqrt{2w+\nu}|0,1,2w+\nu\right) \quad \text{and}$$

$$I_i^{\phi}(w) = \frac{2^w \nu^{\nu/2}}{\sqrt{2\pi}\Gamma(\nu/2)}\left(\frac{1}{d_i+A_i^2+\nu}\right)^{\frac{\nu+2w}{2}} \Gamma\left(\frac{\nu+2w}{2}\right).$$

- *Skew-slash.*

$$I_i^{\Phi}(w) = \frac{2^{w+\nu}\Gamma(w+\nu)}{d_i^{w+\nu}} P_1\left(w+\nu, \frac{d_i}{2}\right) E\left[\Phi(S_i^{1/2}A_i)\right] \quad \text{and}$$

$$I_i^{\phi}(w) = \frac{\nu 2^{w+\nu}\Gamma(w+\nu)}{\sqrt{2\pi}\left(d_i + A_i^2\right)^{w+\nu}} P_1\left(w+\nu, \frac{d_i + A_i^2}{2}\right),$$

where $S_i \sim \text{Gamma}(w+\nu, \frac{d_i}{2})\mathbb{I}_{(0,1)}$.

- *Skew-contaminated normal.*

$$I_i^{\Phi}(w) = \sqrt{2\pi}\left\{\nu\gamma^{w-1/2}\phi_1\left(d_i|0, \frac{1}{\gamma}\right)\Phi\left(\gamma^{1/2}A_i\right) + (1-\nu)\phi_1(d_i|0,1)\Phi(A_i)\right\}$$

and

$$I_i^{\phi}(w) = \nu\gamma^{w-1/2}\phi_1\left(d_i + A_i^2|0, \frac{1}{\gamma}\right) + (1-\nu)\phi_1\left(d_i + A_i^2\right).$$

The derivatives of $\log \mathbf{\Sigma}_i$, d_i, and A_i are direct and are not given here. Asymptotic confidence intervals and tests on the ML estimates can be obtained using this matrix. Thus, if $\mathbf{J} = -\mathbf{L}$ denotes the observed information matrix for the marginal log-likelihood $\ell(\boldsymbol{\theta})$, then asymptotic confidence intervals and hypotheses tests for the parameter $\boldsymbol{\theta} \in \mathbb{R}^q$ are obtained assuming that the MLE $\widehat{\boldsymbol{\theta}}$ has approximately an $\text{N}_q(\boldsymbol{\theta}, \mathbf{J}^{-1})$ distribution. In practice, $\mathbf{J}$ is usually unknown and has to be replaced by the MLE $\widehat{\mathbf{J}}$, that is, the matrix $\widehat{\mathbf{J}}$ evaluated at the MLE $\hat{\boldsymbol{\theta}}$ (see Sect. 2.2). More generally speaking, for models as those in Proposition 3.5, the observed information matrix can be derived from the results given here.

Chapter 4
Univariate Mixture Modeling Using SMSN Distributions

In this chapter we consider a flexible class of probability distributions, convenient for modeling data with skewness behavior, discrepant observations, and population heterogeneity. The elements of this family are convex linear combinations of densities that are scale mixtures of skew-normal distributions. An EM-type algorithm for maximum likelihood estimation is developed and the observed information matrix is obtained. These procedures are discussed with emphasis on finite mixtures of skew-normal, skew-t, skew-slash, and skew-contaminated normal distributions. Essentially, the work is based on Basso et al. (2010), which is an extension of Lin et al. (2007a,b). The proposed EM-type algorithm and methods are implemented in the R package `mixsmsn` (Prates et al. 2013).

4.1 Introduction

The literature on maximum likelihood estimation of the parameters of the normal and Student-t mixture models—hereafter the FM-NOR and the FM-T models, respectively—is very extensive, see McLachlan and Peel (2000) and the references herein, Peel and McLachlan (2000), Nityasuddhi and Böhning (2003), Biernacki and Govaert (2003), and Dias and Wedel (2004), for example. The standard algorithm in this case is the so-called EM (Expectation-Maximization) of Dempster et al. (1977), or maybe some extension like the ECM (Meng and Rubin 1993) or the ECME (Liu and Rubin 1994) algorithms. For a good review, including applications in finite mixture models, see McLachlan and Krishnan (2008).

It is well known that robustness is achieved by modeling the outlier using the Student-t distribution. Finite mixtures of these distributions are useful when there is, besides discrepant observations, unobserved heterogeneity. Here, we suggest a class of models to deal with extra skewness, extending the work of Lin et al. (2007b) and (2007a), where finite mixtures of skew-normal and skew-t distributions are

V. H. Lachos Dávila et al., *Finite Mixture of Skewed Distributions*,
SpringerBriefs in Statistics, https://doi.org/10.1007/978-3-319-98029-4_4

investigated, respectively. The mixture components distributions are assumed to belong to the SMSN family. As commented in Chap. 3, this class contains the entire family of SMN distributions. In addition, the skew-normal and skewed versions of some other classical symmetric distributions are SMSN members: the skew-t, the skew-slash (SSL), and the skew-contaminated normal (SCN), for example. These distributions have heavier tails than the skew-normal (and the normal) one, and thus they seem to be a reasonable choice for robust inference.

The remainder of the chapter is organized as follows. In Sect. 4.2 we propose a finite mixture of scale mixtures of skew-normal distributions (FM-SMSN) and an EM-type algorithm for maximum likelihood estimation. The associated observed information matrix is obtained analytically in Sect. 4.3. In Sect. 4.4 we present a simulation study to show that the proposed models are robust in terms of clustering heterogeneous data and that the maximum likelihood estimates based on the EM-type algorithm do provide good asymptotic properties. Additionally, we report some model selection criteria via simulation. The methodology proposed is illustrated in Sect. 4.5, considering the analysis of a real data set.

4.2 The Proposed Model

The finite mixture of SMSN distributions model (FM-SMSN) is defined by considering a random sample $\mathbf{Y} = (Y_1, \ldots, Y_n)^\top$ from a G-component mixture of univariate SMSN densities given by

$$f(y_i|\boldsymbol{\theta}) = \sum_{j=1}^{G} p_j g(y_i|\boldsymbol{\theta}_j), \; p_j \geq 0, \; \sum_{j=1}^{G} p_j = 1, \; i = 1, \ldots, n, \quad j = 1, \ldots, G, \tag{4.1}$$

where $\boldsymbol{\theta}_j = (\mu_j, \sigma_j^2, \lambda_j, \boldsymbol{\nu}_j^\top)^\top$ is the specific vector of parameters for the component j, $g(\cdot|\boldsymbol{\theta}_j)$ is the SMSN$(\boldsymbol{\theta}_j)$ density, $p_1, \ldots, p_G$ are the mixing probabilities and $\boldsymbol{\theta} = ((p_1, \ldots, p_G)^\top, \boldsymbol{\theta}_1^\top, \ldots, \boldsymbol{\theta}_G^\top)^\top$ is the vector with all parameters. Concerning the parameter $\boldsymbol{\nu}_j$ of the mixing distribution $H(.)$, for $j = 1, \ldots, G$, it is worth noting that it can be a vector of parameters, e.g. the skew-contaminated normal distribution. For computational convenience we assume that $\boldsymbol{\nu}_1 = \ldots = \boldsymbol{\nu}_G = \boldsymbol{\nu}$. This strategy works very well in the empirical studies that we have conducted and greatly simplify the optimization problem.

As in (2.1), for each i and j, consider the latent indicator variable Z_{ij} such that

$$P(Z_{ij} = 1) = 1 - P(Z_{ij} = 0) = p_j, \; \sum_{j=1}^{G} Z_{ij} = 1 \quad \text{and}$$

$$Y_i|Z_{ij} = 1 \sim \text{SMSN}(\boldsymbol{\theta}_j). \tag{4.2}$$

Note that integrating out $\mathbf{Z}_i = (Z_{i1}, \ldots, Z_{iG})^\top$ we obtain the marginal density (4.1). $\mathbf{Z}_1, \ldots, \mathbf{Z}_n$ are independent random vectors, with $\mathbf{Z}_i \sim$ Multinomial$(1; p_1 \ldots, p_G)$.

These latent vectors appear in the hierarchical representation given next, which is used to build the ECME algorithm. From (4.2) along with (3.18)–(3.20), it can be written as

$$Y_i|U_i = u_i, T_i = t_i, Z_{ij} = 1 \sim \mathrm{N}\big(\mu_j + \Delta_j t_i, u_i^{-1}\Gamma_j\big), \quad (4.3)$$

$$T_i|U_i = u_i, Z_{ij} = 1 \sim \mathrm{HN}\big(0, u_i^{-1}\big), \quad (4.4)$$

$$U_i|Z_{ij} = 1 \sim H(u_i; \boldsymbol{\nu}) \quad (4.5)$$

and

$$\mathbf{Z}_i \sim \text{Multinomial}(1; p_1 \ldots, p_G), \quad (4.6)$$

with $i = 1, \ldots, n$ and $j = 1, \ldots, G$, where

$$\Gamma_j = \left(1 - \delta_j^2\right)\sigma_j^2, \quad \Delta_j = \sigma_j\delta_j, \quad \text{and } \delta_j = \frac{\lambda_j}{\sqrt{1+\lambda_j^2}}. \quad (4.7)$$

4.2.1 Maximum Likelihood Estimation via EM Algorithm

In this subsection we show how to implement the EM algorithm for maximum likelihood estimation of the parameters of an FM-SMSN distribution.

By using (4.3)–(4.6), we have that the complete-data log-likelihood function is

$$\ell_c(\boldsymbol{\theta}) = c + \sum_{i=1}^{n}\sum_{j=1}^{G} z_{ij}\Big(\log(p_j) - \frac{1}{2}\log|\Gamma_j| - \frac{u_i}{2\Gamma_j}(y_i - \mu_j - \Delta_j t_i)^2$$
$$+ \log(h(u_i; \boldsymbol{\nu}))\Big),$$

where c is a constant that is independent of the parameter vector $\boldsymbol{\theta}$ and $h(\cdot; \boldsymbol{\nu})$ is the density of U_i. Defining the following quantities

$$\widehat{z}_{ij} = \mathrm{E}\big[Z_{ij}|\widehat{\boldsymbol{\theta}}, y_i\big], \quad \widehat{zu}_{ij} = \mathrm{E}\big[Z_{ij}U_i|\widehat{\boldsymbol{\theta}}, y_i\big], \quad \widehat{zut}_{ij} = \mathrm{E}\big[Z_{ij}U_iT_i|\widehat{\boldsymbol{\theta}}, y_i\big],$$
$$\widehat{zut^2}_{ij} = \mathrm{E}\big[Z_{ij}U_iT_i^2|\widehat{\boldsymbol{\theta}}, y_i\big],$$

and using known properties of conditional expectation, we obtain

$$\widehat{z}_{ij} = \frac{\widehat{p}_j g\big(y_i|\widehat{\boldsymbol{\theta}}_j\big)}{\sum_{j=1}^{G} \widehat{p}_j g\big(y_i|\widehat{\boldsymbol{\theta}}_j\big)}, \tag{4.8}$$
$$\widehat{zu}_{ij} = \widehat{z}_{ij}\widehat{u}_{ij}, \quad \widehat{zut}_{ij} = \widehat{z}_{ij}\big(\widehat{u}_{ij}\widehat{m}_{ij} + \widehat{M}_j\widehat{\eta}_{ij}\big),$$
$$\widehat{zut^2}_{ij} = \widehat{z}_{ij}\big(\widehat{u}_{ij}\widehat{m}^2_{ij} + \widehat{M}^2_j + \widehat{M}_j\widehat{m}_{ij}\widehat{\eta}_{ij}\big),$$

where

$$\widehat{\eta}_{ij} = E\left[U_i^{1/2} W_{\Phi_1}\left(\frac{U_i^{1/2}\widehat{m}_{ij}}{\widehat{M}_j}\right) \mid \widehat{\boldsymbol{\theta}}, y_i, Z_{ij} = 1\right],$$

$$\widehat{M}^2_j = \frac{\widehat{\Gamma}_j}{\widehat{\Gamma}_j + \widehat{\Delta}^2_j}, \quad \widehat{m}_{ij} = \frac{\widehat{\Delta}_j}{\widehat{\Gamma}_j + \widehat{\Delta}^2_j}(y_i - \widehat{\mu}_j)$$

and

$$\widehat{u}_{ij} = E\big[U_i|\widehat{\boldsymbol{\theta}}, y_i, Z_{ij} = 1\big], \qquad i = 1, \ldots, n, \quad j = 1, \ldots, G.$$

Once again, in each step, the conditional expectations $\widehat{u}_{ij}$ and $\widehat{\eta}_{ij}$ can be easily derived from the results given in Sect. 3.3.1. Thus, the Q-function is given by

$$\begin{aligned}
Q(\boldsymbol{\theta}|\widehat{\boldsymbol{\theta}}^{(k)}) = c + \sum_{i=1}^{n}\sum_{j=1}^{G}\Bigg(\widehat{z}_{ij}^{(k+1)}\left(\log(p_j) - \frac{1}{2}\log|\Gamma_j|\right)\\
-\frac{1}{2\Gamma_j}\left(\widehat{u}_{ij}^{(k+1)}(y_i - \mu_j)^2\right.\\
\left.-2(y_i - \mu_j)\Delta_j\widehat{zut}_{ij}^{(k+1)} + \Delta_j^2\widehat{zut^2}_{ij}^{(k+1)}\right)\\
+E\left[Z_{ij}\log(h(U_i;\boldsymbol{\nu}))|\widehat{\boldsymbol{\theta}}^{(k)}, y_i\right]\Bigg).
\end{aligned}$$

When the M-step turns out to be analytically intractable, it can be replaced with a sequence of conditional maximization (CM) steps. The resulting procedure is known as the ECM algorithm. The ECME algorithm, a faster extension of EM and ECM, is obtained by maximizing the constrained Q-function with some CM-steps that maximize the corresponding constrained actual marginal likelihood function, called CML-steps. Next, we describe this EM-type algorithm (ECME) for maximum likelihood estimation of the parameters of the FM-SMSN.

E-Step Given a current estimate $\widehat{\boldsymbol{\theta}}^{(k)}$, compute $\widehat{z}_{ij}$, $\widehat{zu}_{ij}$, $\widehat{zut}_{ij}$, $\widehat{zut^2}_{ij}$, for $i = 1, \ldots, n$ and $j = 1, \ldots, G$.

CM-Steps Update $\widehat{\boldsymbol{\theta}}^{(k)}$ by maximizing $Q(\boldsymbol{\theta}|\widehat{\boldsymbol{\theta}}^{(k)}) = E[\ell_c(\boldsymbol{\theta})|\mathbf{y}, \widehat{\boldsymbol{\theta}}^{(k)}]$ over $\boldsymbol{\theta}$, which leads to the following closed form expressions:

$$\widehat{p}_j^{(k+1)} = n^{-1}\sum_{i=1}^{n}\widehat{z}_{ij}^{(k+1)},$$

$$\widehat{\mu}_j^{(k+1)} = \sum_{i=1}^{n}\left(\widehat{zu}_{ij}^{(k+1)}y_i - \widehat{\Delta}_j^{(k)}\widehat{zut}_{ij}^{(k+1)}\right)\Big/\sum_{i=1}^{n}\widehat{zu}_{ij}^{(k+1)},$$

$$\widehat{\Delta}_j^{(k+1)} = \sum_{i=1}^{n}\left(y_i - \widehat{\mu}_j^{(k+1)}\right)\widehat{zut}_{ij}^{(k+1)}\Big/\sum_{i=1}^{n}\widehat{zut2}_{ij}^{(k+1)}, \quad \text{and}$$

$$\widehat{\Gamma}_j^{(k+1)} = \frac{\sum_{i=1}^{n}\left(\widehat{zu}_{ij}^{(k+1)}\left(y_i - \widehat{\mu}_j^{(k+1)}\right)^2 - 2\left(y_i - \widehat{\mu}_j^{(k+1)}\right)\widehat{\Delta}_j^{(k+1)}\widehat{zut}_{ij}^{(k+1)} + \left(\widehat{\Delta}_j^2\right)^{(k+1)}\widehat{zut2}_{ij}^{(k+1)}\right)}{\sum_{i=1}^{n}\widehat{z}_{ij}^{(k+1)}}.$$

CML-Step Update $\widehat{\boldsymbol{\nu}}^{(k)}$ by maximizing the actual marginal log-likelihood function, obtaining

$$\widehat{\boldsymbol{\nu}}^{(k+1)} = \operatorname{argmax}_{\boldsymbol{\nu}}\sum_{i=1}^{n}\log\left(\sum_{j=1}^{G}\widehat{p}_j^{(k+1)}g\left(y_i|\widehat{\mu}_j^{(k+1)}, \widehat{\sigma}_j^{2(k+1)}, \widehat{\lambda}_j^{(k+1)}, \boldsymbol{\nu}\right)\right). \tag{4.9}$$

This process is iterated until a suitable convergence rule is satisfied, e.g. if $||\widehat{\boldsymbol{\theta}}^{(k+1)} - \widehat{\boldsymbol{\theta}}^{(k)}||$ is sufficiently small, or until some distance involving two successive evaluations of the actual log-likelihood $\ell(\boldsymbol{\theta})$, like $||\ell(\widehat{\boldsymbol{\theta}}^{(k+1)}) - \ell(\widehat{\boldsymbol{\theta}}^{(k)})||$ or $||\ell(\widehat{\boldsymbol{\theta}}^{(k+1)})/\ell(\widehat{\boldsymbol{\theta}}^{(k)}) - 1||$, is small enough. See Dias and Wedel (2004) for a discussion in the context of mixtures of univariate normal distributions.

An important feature of this algorithm is that, for skew-normal data, that is, $U_i = 1$, for $i, \ldots, n$, we have explicit solutions for the M-step—see the CM-steps above. Also, for general U_i, numerical methods, like the Newton's Method, are needed for solving Eq. (4.9). On the other hand, the algorithms proposed by Lin et al. (2007b) (skew-normal case) and Lin et al. (2007a) (skew-t case) do not produce closed form expressions to obtain current estimates for the skewness parameter. In our case, parameterization (4.7) allows us to circumvent this problem easily.

An usual criticism is that EM-type procedures tend to get stuck in local modes. A convenient way to avoid such limitations is to try several EM iterations with a variety of starting values. If there exist several modes, one can find the global mode by comparing their relative masses and log-likelihood values.

4.2.2 Notes on Implementation

It is well known that mixture models may provide a multimodal log-likelihood function. In this sense, the method of maximum likelihood estimation through EM algorithm may not give maximum global solutions if the starting values are far from the real parameter values. Thus, the choice of starting values for the EM algorithm in the mixture context plays a big role in parameter estimation. In our examples and simulation studies we consider the following procedure for the FM-SMSN model

- Partition the sample into G groups using the K-means clustering algorithm (Hartigan and Wong 1979);
- Compute the proportion of data points belonging to the same cluster j, say $\widehat{p}_j^{(0)}$, $j = 1, \ldots, G$. This is the initial value for p_j;
- For each group j, compute the initial values $\widehat{\mu}_j^{(0)}$, $\widehat{\sigma}_j^{2(0)}$, and $\widehat{\lambda}_j^{(0)}$ using the following method of moments (see Proposition 3.7). First, we consider $\boldsymbol{\nu}$ fixed. Let us denote the method of moments estimator of $\boldsymbol{\theta} = (\mu, \sigma^2, \delta)^\top$ by $\widetilde{\boldsymbol{\theta}} = (\widetilde{\mu}, \widetilde{\sigma}^2, \widetilde{\delta})^\top$, where $\delta = \lambda/\sqrt{1+\lambda^2}$. The estimator is given by

$$M_3\left(k_2 - \frac{2}{\pi}k_1^2\widetilde{\delta}^2\right)^{3/2} = (M_2)^{3/2}(a_1 + a_2\widetilde{\delta}^2)\widetilde{\delta},$$

$$\widetilde{\sigma}^2 = \frac{M_2}{\left(k_2 - \frac{2}{\pi}k_1^2\widetilde{\delta}^2\right)}$$

and

$$\widetilde{\mu} = M_1 - k_1\sqrt{\frac{2}{\pi}}\widetilde{\sigma}\widetilde{\delta},$$

where $M_1 = \frac{1}{n}\sum_{i=1}^n y_i$, $M_2 = \frac{1}{n}\sum_{i=1}^n (y_i - \overline{y})^2$, $M_3 = \frac{1}{n}\sum_{i=1}^n (y_i - \overline{y})^3$, $k_m = E(U^{-m/2})$, $a_1 = 3(2/\pi)^{1/2}(k_3 - k_1k_2)$, $a_2 = 2(2/\pi)^{3/2}k_1^3 - (2/\pi)k_3$ and U is the scale factor of $Y \sim SMSN_p(\mu, \sigma^2, \lambda; H)$. Although we do not have a closed form expression for $\widetilde{\delta}$, we can apply some computational procedures (such as the Newton-Raphson method) to obtain numerical solutions. However, when $U = 1$, the equations above reduce to the equations obtained by Arnold et al. (1993); see also Lin et al. (2007b).

The range for the skewness coefficient γ_1 of the SN distribution is approximately $(-0.9953, 0.9953)$ (Azzalini 2005). But the method of moments can produce an initial value $\widehat{\gamma}_1^{(0)}$ that is not in this interval. In this case, we use as starting points the values -0.99 (if $\widehat{\gamma}_1^{(0)} \leq -0.9953$) or 0.99 (if $\widehat{\gamma}_1^{(0)} \geq 0.9953$).

When modeling using the FM-ST, FM-SCN or the FM-SSL models we adopt the following strategy:

- Obtain initial values via method of moments for the FM-SN model, as described above;

- Perform maximum likelihood estimation of the parameters of the FM-SN model via ECME algorithm;
- Use the ECME estimates of the location, scale, and skewness parameters of the FM-SN model as initial values for the corresponding FM-ST and FM-SCN parameters;
- The starting values for ν are taken close to 10 in the FM-ST case and $\boldsymbol{\nu} = (0.5, 0.5)^\top$ in the FM-SCN case. For the FM-SSL model, the starting value was fixed as the ECME estimate of ν for the FM-ST model.

4.3 The Observed Information Matrix

It is well known that, under some regularity conditions, the covariance matrix of the maximum likelihood estimates $\widehat{\boldsymbol{\theta}}$ can be approximated by $\mathbf{J}_o(\widehat{\boldsymbol{\theta}}|\mathbf{Y})^{-1}/n$, where $\mathbf{J}_o(\widehat{\boldsymbol{\theta}}|\mathbf{Y})^{-1}$ is the inverse of observed information matrix, see (2.6). By (2.7), we evaluate

$$\mathbf{J}_o\big(\widehat{\boldsymbol{\theta}}|\mathbf{Y}\big) = \sum_{i=1}^{n} \widehat{\mathbf{s}}_i \widehat{\mathbf{s}}_i^\top, \tag{4.10}$$

where

$$\widehat{\mathbf{s}}_i = \frac{\partial \left(\log \sum_{j=1}^{G} p_j g(y_i|\boldsymbol{\theta}_j)\right)}{\partial \boldsymbol{\theta}} \Big|_{\boldsymbol{\theta}=\widehat{\boldsymbol{\theta}}} .$$

We consider now the vector $\widehat{\mathbf{s}}_i$ which is partitioned into components corresponding to all the parameters in $\boldsymbol{\theta}$ as

$$\widehat{\mathbf{s}}_i = \left(\widehat{s}_{i,p_1}, \ldots, \widehat{s}_{i,p_{G-1}}, \widehat{s}_{i,\mu_1}, \ldots, \widehat{s}_{i,\mu_G}, \widehat{s}_{i,\sigma_1^2}, \ldots, \widehat{s}_{i,\sigma_G^2}, \widehat{s}_{i,\lambda_1}, \ldots, \widehat{s}_{i,\lambda_G}, \widehat{s}_{i,\boldsymbol{\nu}}\right)^\top,$$

where the coordinate elements in $\widehat{\mathbf{s}}_i$ are given by

$$\widehat{s}_{i,p_r} = \frac{g(y_i|\boldsymbol{\theta}_r) - g(y_i|\boldsymbol{\theta}_G)}{f(y_i|\boldsymbol{\theta})}, \quad \widehat{s}_{i,\mu_r} = \frac{p_r D_{\mu_r}(g(y_i|\boldsymbol{\theta}_r))}{f(y_i|\boldsymbol{\theta})},$$

$$\widehat{s}_{i,\sigma_r^2} = \frac{p_r D_{\sigma_r^2}(g(y_i|\boldsymbol{\theta}_r))}{f(y_i|\boldsymbol{\theta})}, \quad \widehat{s}_{i,\lambda_r} = \frac{p_r D_{\lambda_r}(g(y_i|\boldsymbol{\theta}_r))}{f(y_i|\boldsymbol{\theta})}$$

and

$$\widehat{s}_{i,\boldsymbol{\nu}} = \frac{\sum_{j=1}^{G} p_j D_{\boldsymbol{\nu}}(g(y_i|\boldsymbol{\theta}_r))}{f(y_i|\boldsymbol{\theta})},$$

where

$$D_{\mu_r}(g(y_i|\boldsymbol{\theta}_r)) = \frac{\partial}{\partial \mu_r}(g(y_i|\boldsymbol{\theta}_r))$$

and $D_{\sigma_r^2}$, D_{λ_r}, and $D_{\boldsymbol{\nu}}$ are defined by analogy, $r = 1, \ldots, G$. Note that $D_{\boldsymbol{\nu}}(g(y_i|\boldsymbol{\theta}_r))$ must be obtained for each particular case (i.e., ST, SSL, and SCN). Let us define

$$I_{ir}^{\Phi}(w) = \int_0^{\infty} u_i^w \exp\left\{-\frac{1}{2}u_i d_{ir}\right\} \Phi\left(u_i^{1/2} A_{ir}\right) dH(u_i)$$

and

$$I_{ir}^{\phi}(w) = \int_0^{\infty} u_i^w \exp\left\{-\frac{1}{2}u_i d_{ir}\right\} \phi\left(u_i^{1/2} (A_{ir})^{1/2}\right) dH(u_i),$$

where

$$d_{ir} = \frac{(y_i - \mu_r)^2}{\sigma_r^2} \quad \text{and} \quad A_{ir} = \lambda_r \frac{(y_i - \mu_r)}{\sigma_r}, \quad i = 1, \ldots, n, \quad r = 1, \ldots, G.$$

After some algebraic manipulation, we obtain

$$D_{\mu_r}(g(y_i|\boldsymbol{\theta}_r)) = \frac{2}{\sqrt{2\pi\sigma_r^2}}\left[-\sigma_r^{-1}\lambda_r I_{ir}^{\phi}(1) + \frac{(y_i - \mu_r)}{\sigma_r^2} I_{ir}^{\Phi}(3/2)\right],$$

$$D_{\sigma_r^2}(g(y_i|\boldsymbol{\theta}_r)) = \frac{2}{\sqrt{2\pi}}\left[-\frac{1}{2}\sigma_r^{-3} I_{ir}^{\Phi}(1/2) + (y_i - \mu_r)^2 \sigma_r^{-4} I_{ir}^{\Phi}(3/2)\right.$$
$$\left. -\lambda_r \sigma_r^{-3}(y_i - \mu_r) I_{ir}^{\phi}(1)\right],$$

and

$$D_{\lambda_r}(g(y_i|\boldsymbol{\theta}_r)) = \frac{2}{\sqrt{2\pi\sigma_r^2}}\sigma_r^{-1}(y_i - \mu_r) I_{ir}^{\phi}(1).$$

Lachos et al. (2010) have shown that, for each distribution considered in this work, we have closed form expressions for the quantities $I_{ir}^{\Phi}(w)$, $I_{ir}^{\phi}(w)$ and $D_{\boldsymbol{\nu}}(g(y_i|\boldsymbol{\theta}_r))$, $i = 1, \ldots, n$, $r = 1, \ldots, G$, as follows:

4.3.1 The Skew-t Distribution

$$I_{ir}^{\Phi}(w) = \frac{2^w \nu^{\nu/2}\Gamma(w+\nu/2)}{\sqrt{2\pi}\Gamma(\nu/2)(\nu+d_{ir})^{\nu/2+w}} T\left(\frac{A_{ir}}{(d_{ir}+\nu)^{1/2}}\sqrt{2w+\nu}; 2w+\nu\right),$$

$$I_{ir}^{\phi}(w) = \frac{2^w \nu^{\nu/2}}{\sqrt{2\pi}\Gamma(\nu/2)} \left(\frac{1}{d_{ir}+A_{ir}^2+\nu}\right)^{\frac{\nu+2w}{2}} \Gamma\left(\frac{\nu+2w}{2}\right),$$

and

$$D_\nu(g(y_i|\boldsymbol{\theta}_r)) = \frac{1}{\sqrt{2\pi\sigma_r^2}}\Big[(\log(\boldsymbol{\nu}/2)+1+DG(\boldsymbol{\nu}/2)I_{ir}^{\Phi}(1/2) - I_{ir}^{\Phi}(3/2)$$
$$+\int_0^\infty u^{1/2}\log(u)\exp(-u\, d_{ir}/2)\Phi(u^{1/2}A_{ir})h(u;\boldsymbol{\nu})du\Big].$$

4.3.2 The Skew-Slash Distribution

$$I_{ir}^{\Phi}(w) = \frac{2^{2+\nu}\Gamma(w+\nu)}{d_{ir}^{w+\nu}} P_1(w+\nu, d_{ir}/2)E\big[\Phi(S_{ir}^{1/2})A_{ir}\big],$$

$$I_{ir}^{\phi}(w) = \frac{\nu 2^{w+\nu}\Gamma(w+\nu)}{\sqrt{2\pi}(d_{ir}+A_{ir}^2)^{w+\nu}} P_1\left(w+\nu, \frac{d_{ir}+A_{ir}^2}{2}\right),$$

where $S_{ir} \sim Gamma(w+\nu, d_{ir}/2)I_{(0,1)}$ and

$$D_\nu(g(y_i|\boldsymbol{\theta}_r)) = 2\int_0^1 u^{\nu-1}[1+\nu\log(u_i)]\phi\big(y_i;\mu_r, u^{-1}\sigma_r^2\big)\Phi\big(u^{1/2}A_{ir}\big)du_i.$$

4.3.3 The Skew-Contaminated Normal Distribution

$$I_{ir}^{\Phi}(w) = \sqrt{2\pi}\Big\{\nu\gamma^{w-1/2}\phi\Big(\sqrt{d_{ir}}; 0, \frac{1}{\gamma}\Big)\Phi(\gamma^{1/2}A_{ir})$$
$$+(1-\nu)\phi(\sqrt{d_{ir}})\Phi(A_{ir})\Big\},$$

$$I_{ir}^{\phi}(w) = \nu\gamma^{w-1/2}\phi\left((d_{ir}+A_{ir}^2)^{1/2}; 0, \frac{1}{\gamma}\right)$$

$$+(1-\nu)\phi\left(\left(d_{ir}+A_{ir}^2\right)^{1/2};0,1\right),$$

$$D_\nu(g(y_i;\boldsymbol{\theta}_r)) = 2\left(\phi\left(y_i;\mu_r,\gamma^{-1}\sigma_r^2\right)\Phi\left(\gamma^{1/2}A_{ir}\right) - g\left(y_i|\mu_r,\sigma_r^2\right)\Phi(A_{ir})\right)$$

and

$$\begin{aligned}D_\gamma(g(y_i|\boldsymbol{\theta}_r)) = &\frac{\nu}{\sqrt{2\pi\sigma^2}}\gamma^{1/2}\exp(-\gamma d_{ir}/2)\Big[\gamma^{-1}\Phi\left(\gamma^{1/2}A_{ir}\right)\\ &+\phi\left(\gamma^{-1/2}A_{ir}\right)A_{ir}\gamma^{-1/2}\\ &-\Phi(\gamma^{1/2}A_{ir})d_{ir}\Big].\end{aligned}$$

The information-based approximation (4.10) is asymptotically applicable. However, it may not be reliable unless the sample size is large. In practice, it is common to perform the bootstrap approach (Efron and Tibshirani 1986) to obtain an alternative estimate of the covariance matrix of $\widehat{\boldsymbol{\theta}}$. The bootstrap method may provide more accurate standard error estimates than (4.10). However, it requires an enormous amount of computation.

4.4 Simulation Studies

In order to examine the performance of the proposed method, we present some simulation studies. The first simulation study shows that the underlying FM-SMSN models are robust in the ability to cluster heterogeneous data. The second simulation study shows that our proposed ECME algorithm estimates do provide good asymptotic properties. In the third study we compare some model selection criteria.

4.4.1 Study 1: Clustering

First, we investigate the ability of the FM-SMSN models in clustering observations, that is, allocate them into groups of observations that are similar in some sense. We know that each data point belongs to one of G heterogeneous populations, but we do not know how to discriminate between them. Modeling by mixture models allows clustering of the data in terms of the estimated (posterior) probability that a single point belongs to a given group.

A lot of work in model-based clustering has been done using finite mixtures of normal distributions. As the posterior probabilities $\widehat{z}_{ij}$—see (4.8)—can be highly influenced by atypical observations, there were efforts to develop robust alternatives, like mixtures of Student-t distributions (see McLachlan and Peel (1998) and the references herein). Our idea is to extend the flexibility of these models, by including possible skewness of the related components.

We generated 500 samples from a mixture of two SMSN densities and, for each sample, proceeded clustering ignoring the known true classification. The FM-SMSN models were fitted using the algorithm described in Sect. 4.2.1, in order to obtain the estimate of the posterior probability that an observation y_i belongs to the jth component of the mixture, $\widehat{z}_{ij}$. Then, the threshold value 0.5 was used to allocate the observation to some specific component. For sample l, $l = 1, \ldots, 500$, we compute the rate r_l, the number of correct allocations divided by the sample size n. When fitting the FM-SSL model, the parameter ν was considered known and we fixed $\nu = 2$. We have not considered modeling using the FM-SSL model with unknown ν because, in this case, the algorithm is very time-consuming.

We fixed the parameter values at $\mu_1 = 15$, $\mu_2 = 20$, $\sigma_1^2 = 20$, $\sigma_2^2 = 16$, $\lambda_1 = 6$, $\lambda_2 = -4$, $p_1 = 0.8$, and $\nu = 3$. For the SCN case we fixed $(\nu_1, \gamma_1) = (\nu_2, \gamma_2) = (0.2, 0.2)$. The sample sizes considered were $n = 100, 500, 1000$.

In Fig. 4.1a we plot a histogram of one sample taken from an FM-ST population with $n = 500$. It shows a mixture of skew-t observations that overlap largely, meaning that the data in the components are poorly separated. Note that, although we have a two-component mixture, the histogram need not to be bimodal.

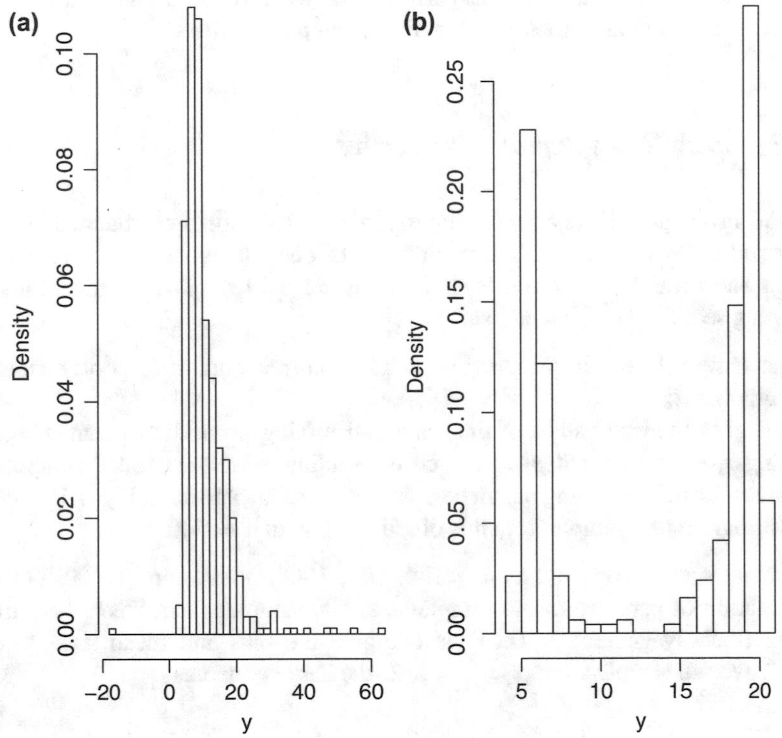

Fig. 4.1 Artificial FM-ST data ($n = 500$) with two components: (**a**) poorly separated components; (**b**) well-separated components

Table 4.1 Mean right allocations rates for fitted FM-SMSN models

True model	Sample size	Fitted model FM-NOR	FM-SN	FM-ST	FM-SCN	FM-SSL
FM-ST	100	0.4102	0.6825	0.7872	0.7879	0.7705
	500	0.3067	0.7521	0.8369	0.8340	0.8329
	1000	0.2942	0.7834	0.8381	0.8375	0.8361
FM-SCN	100	0.5601	0.6967	0.7783	0.7778	0.7686
	500	0.6072	0.7904	0.8324	0.8340	0.8323
	1000	0.6406	0.8139	0.8349	0.8346	0.8358
FM-SSL	100	0.5765	0.7602	0.7755	0.7669	0.7562
	500	0.6162	0.8216	0.8336	0.8341	0.8324
	1000	0.6287	0.8340	0.8336	0.8327	0.8341

Table 4.1 shows the mean value of the correct allocations rates, that is, $(1/500)\sum_{l=1}^{500} r_l$. Comparing with the results for the FM-NOR model, we see that modeling using the FM-SN, FM-ST, FM-SCN, or FM-SSL distributions represents a substantial improvement in the outright clustering. Also, the FM-ST, FM-SCN and FM-SSL models have a better performance when the true model is FM-ST or FM-SCN, showing their robustness to discrepant observations.

4.4.2 *Study 2: Asymptotic Properties*

We now investigate some asymptotic properties of the estimates obtained using the suggested ECME algorithm. The main focus of our interest are on the evaluations of bias and mean square error. Here we consider only the FM-ST model and the following sets of true parameter values:

1. The same set used in the previous section, corresponding to poorly separated components;
2. Changing the true values of the scale and mixing proportion parameters, now using $\sigma_1 = \sigma_2 = 1$ and $p_1 = 0.4$, corresponding to well-separated components. Values for the remaining parameters are the same as before. In Fig. 4.1b we have a histogram of a sample from this distribution with $n = 500$.

Sample sizes were fixed as n =100, 500, 1000, 5000, and 10,000. For each combination of parameters and sample size, 500 samples from the FM-ST model were artificially generated. Then we compute the bias and mean squared error (MSE) over all samples. For $\mu_j,\ \ j = 1, 2$, they are defined as

$$\text{bias} = \frac{1}{500}\sum_{i=1}^{500} \widehat{\mu}_j^{(i)} - \mu_j \quad \text{and} \quad \text{MSE} = \frac{1}{500}\sum_{i=1}^{500} \left(\widehat{\mu}_j^{(i)} - \mu_j\right)^2,$$

respectively, where $\widehat{\mu}_j^{(i)}$ is the ECME estimate of μ_j when the data is sample i. Definitions for the other parameters are obtained by analogy.

Tables 4.2 and 4.3 present the results for the poorly (PS) and well-separated (WS) cases, respectively, with $\nu = 3$ as a reference value, meanwhile Figs. 4.2 and 4.3 show a graphical representation only for the bias in the PS and WS case, respectively. We can see the following patterns of convergence to zero

1. *The WS case*. With a sample size greater than 100, the MSE of location parameters has value less than 0.007, the MSE of scales is less than 0.1, and the MSE of proportions is less than 0.004. When the sample size is greater than 500, the MSE for degrees of freedom is less than 0.4. These results are satisfactory, from our point of view. The worst case scenario seems to happen while estimating the skewness parameters, perhaps due to the well-known inferential problems related to the skewness parameter in skew-normal models; see DiCiccio and Monti (2004), or maybe a sample size greater than 1000 is needed to obtain a reasonably pattern of convergence.
2. *The PS case*. Here, reasonably small bias and MSE in mean and mixing proportions seem to occur for the sample size greater than 500. For the skewness, scale and degrees of freedom parameters, convergence to zero seems to be slower, and satisfactory values of MSE seem to occur when n is greater than 1000.

As a general rule, we can say that bias and MSE tend to approach to zero when the sample size is increasing. These results agree with the remarks made by Nityasuddhi and Böhning (2003), when studying the asymptotic properties of the EM estimates for the FM-NOR model.

We have also considered several values for the degrees of freedom parameter ν (equal to 3, 6, 10, 15, 20, 30, and 50), in order to evaluate the effect of ν on the estimation of other parameters, notably the scale parameter σ_j^2 and the skewness parameter λ_j. We did not find any influence of ν parameter, at least for the set of parameters used in our simulation study. The bias and MSE values were close to each other, suggesting that they are independent of the value of ν.

4.4.3 Study 3: Model Selection

Here we compare the ability of some classical procedures in choosing between the underlying FM-SMSN models. We fixed the number of components ($G = 2$), sample size ($n = 1000$), and parameter values ($\mu_1 = 20$, $\mu_2 = 30$, $\sigma_1^2 = 15$, $\sigma_2^2 = 40$, $\lambda_1 = 2$, $\lambda_2 = 10$ and $p_1 = 0.6$). Several values for the degrees of freedom parameter ν (equal to 3, 6, 10, 15 and 30) were taken into account. Then, for each combination value of the parameters, 500 samples from a mixture of skew-t densities were artificially generated and, for each sample, we fitted the FM-SN and the FM-ST models. For each fitted model, we computed the Akaike Information Criterion (AIC) (Akaike 1974), the Bayesian Information Criterion (BIC) (Schwarz 1978), the Efficient Determination Criterion (EDC) (Bai et al.

Table 4.2 Bias and mean squared errors for ECME estimates—poorly separated components

		Sample size				
Measure	Parameter	100	500	1000	5000	10,000
Bias	μ_1	3.626685e−02	9.553629e−04	2.251980e−04	−6.480655e−04	−3.259887e−04
	μ_2	−4.043036e−01	−2.082871e−02	−3.225519e−03	−6.226229e−03	−2.37579e−03
	σ_1^2	−5.192698e−01	−3.552685e−02	−6.928553e−03	2.437042e−05	−1.77739e−03
	σ_2^2	5.172681e−01	−6.393652e−02	9.639911e−02	7.684399e−03	3.255335e−03
	λ_1	2.962971e+00	1.799639e−01	5.203251e−02	4.408876e−03	4.129488e−04
	λ_2	−1.221872e+01	−2.345765e−01	−1.041270e−01	−2.643574e−03	−3.593367e−03
	ν	1.178223e+02	1.442717e−01	5.591489e−02	1.192845e−02	4.705524e−03
	p_1	−1.899612e−02	−2.633289e−03	−1.884522e−05	3.049117e−07	1.450857e−04
MSE	μ_1	1.151169e−01	9.618573e−03	3.961588e−03	2.836060e−04	7.941788e−05
	μ_2	2.057845e+00	1.306358e−01	4.897538e−02	3.154556e−03	9.266971e−05
	σ_1^2	1.833444e+01	1.107149e+00	2.085420e−01	3.284945e−03	5.445568e−04
	σ_2^2	1.862787e+02	1.571325e+01	4.580214e+00	6.833315e−02	1.346153e−02
	λ_1	1.157501e+02	9.825899e−01	2.416234e−01	8.612938e−03	1.380906e−03
	λ_2	7.212604e+02	2.469349e+00	5.175716e−01	8.273690e−03	1.710742e−03
	ν	1.014661e+03	5.657795e−01	1.021304e−01	1.472001e−02	6.089940e−03
	p_1	7.401136e−03	7.574217e−04	3.783682e−04	6.581538e−05	2.512335e−05

Table 4.3 Bias and mean squared errors for ECME estimates—well-separated components

Measure	Parameter	Sample size				
		100	500	1000	5000	10,000
Bias	μ_1	2.240432e−02	1.387814e−03	1.685946e−03	4.182902e−05	2.235176e−05
	μ_2	−1.153799e−02	−4.052004e−03	−1.395336e−03	7.981414e−05	−4.667282e−05
	σ_1^2	1.080980e−02	9.245055e−05	6.969676e−04	−4.585860e−05	−9.148042e−06
	σ_2^2	1.493537e−02	−1.407618e−03	2.249074e−03	−2.232164e−04	7.266806e−05
	λ_1	4.044328e+02	2.150470e+00	4.582539e−01	6.167612e−03	1.653220e−03
	λ_2	−1.431243e+01	−3.589517e−01	−1.137305e−01	−1.626848e−02	2.566557e−03
	ν	2.527001e+00	1.765753e−01	4.866826e−02	1.145722e−02	−1.965416e−03
	p_1	5.931726e−04	5.989383e−04	1.387312e−03	−5.946862e−04	−8.035652e−05
MSE	μ_1	5.235930e−03	4.353205e−04	1.729061e−04	7.793829e−06	1.072331e−06
	μ_2	6.361194e−03	7.572480e−04	2.695497e−04	1.874958e−05	5.167974e−06
	σ_1^2	3.956735e−02	1.528215e−03	1.997454e−04	1.720467e−06	1.546036e−07
	σ_2^2	9.320955e−02	5.710687e−03	1.208212e−03	1.520323e−05	2.486816e−06
	λ_1	4.231106e+03	5.384741e+01	7.080843e+00	1.445613e−01	1.548913e−02
	λ_2	1.402899e+03	4.138201e+00	8.713269e−01	3.303539e−02	4.560911e−03
	ν	1.420523e+02	3.322731e−01	8.918025e−02	1.585834e−02	8.78927e−03
	p_1	3.077124e−03	5.033739e−04	2.744831e−04	4.742073e−05	2.37786e−05

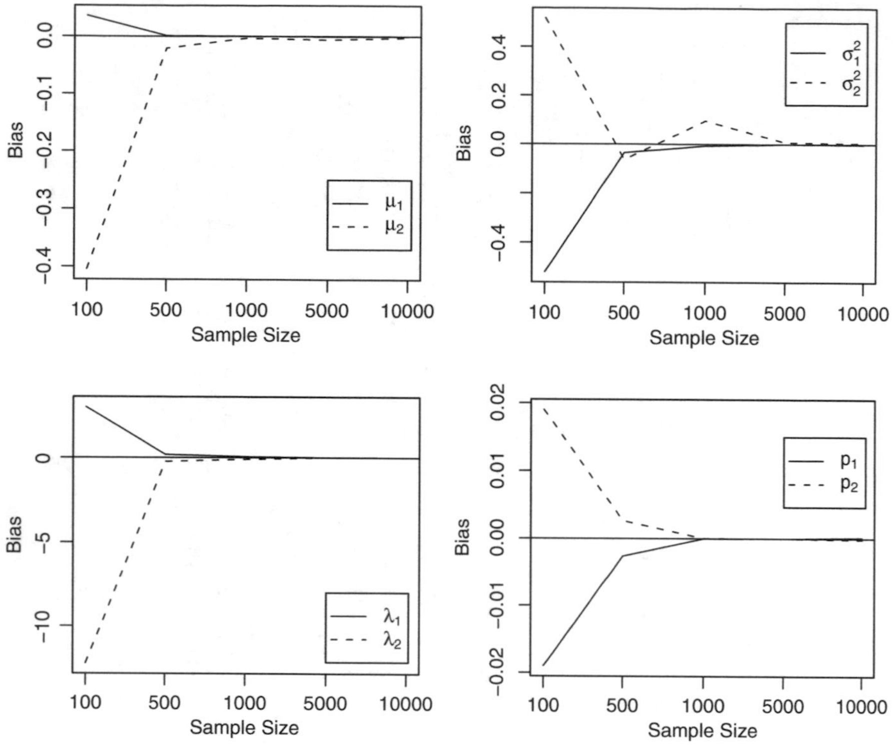

Fig. 4.2 Bias in ECME estimates—poorly separated components

1989), and the Integrated Completed Likelihood Criterion (ICL) (Biernacki et al. 2000). AIC, BIC, and EDC have the form

$$-2\ell(\widehat{\boldsymbol{\theta}}) + \gamma c_n, \tag{4.11}$$

where $\ell(\cdot)$ is the actual log-likelihood, γ is the number of free parameters that have to be estimated under the model, and the penalty term c_n is a convenient sequence of positive numbers. We have $c_n = 2$ for AIC and $c_n = \log(n)$ for BIC. For the EDC criterion, c_n is chosen so that it satisfies the conditions $c_n/n \to 0$ and $c_n/(\log\log n) \to 0$ when $n \to \infty$. Here we use $c_n = 0.2\sqrt{n}$, a proposal that was considered in Bai et al. (1989). The ICL is defined as

$$-2\ell^*(\widehat{\boldsymbol{\theta}}) + \gamma \log(n),$$

where $\ell^*(\cdot)$ is the integrated log-likelihood of the sample and the indicator latent variables—see (4.2), given by

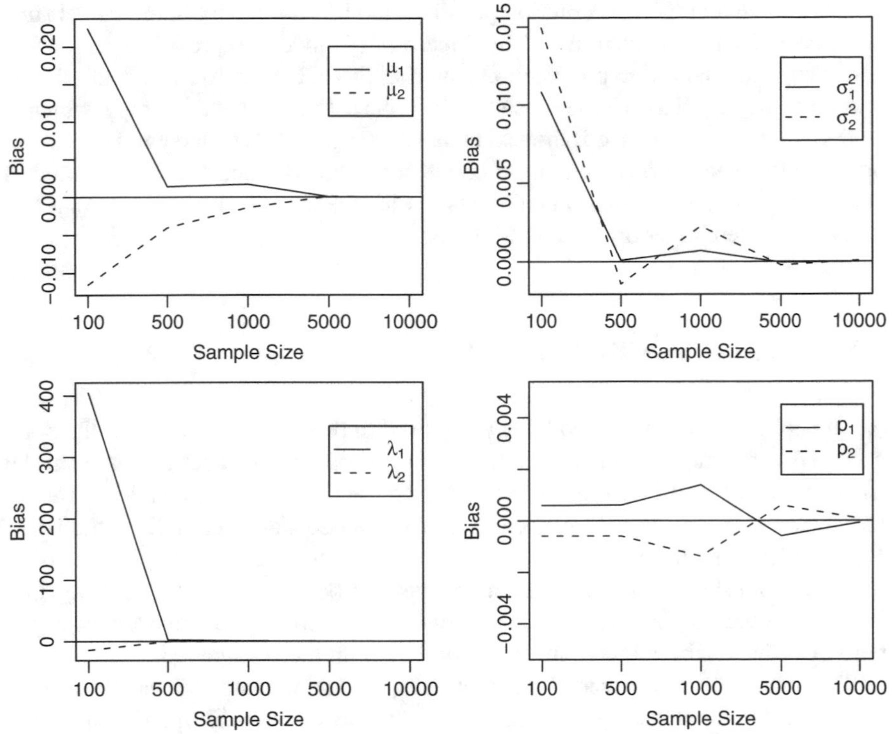

Fig. 4.3 Bias in ECME estimates—well-separated components

Table 4.4 Number of times (out of 500) the true model is chosen using different criteria

	Degrees of freedom				
Criterion	3	6	10	15	30
AIC	500	488	424	330	139
BIC	500	469	279	135	22
EDC	500	475	296	145	33
ICL	438	93	7	1	0

$$\ell^*(\widehat{\boldsymbol{\theta}}) = \sum_{i=1}^{g} \sum_{j \in \mathscr{C}_i} \log\left(\widehat{p}_i g\left(y_j | \widehat{\boldsymbol{\theta}}_i\right)\right),$$

where $\mathscr{C}_i$ is a set of indexes defined as: j belongs to $\mathscr{C}_i$ if, and only if, the observation y_j is allocated to component i by the clustering method presented in Sect. 4.4.1.

Table 4.4 shows the number of times the true model is chosen for each combination of criterion and degrees of freedom. When ν is 3 or 6, all the criteria have a satisfactory behavior except ICL, which has maintained a low performance for all remaining values of ν. For $\nu = 10$, 15, and 30, AIC has the best behavior.

It is known that the ICL criterion penalizes model complexity in the model (like AIC and BIC) and the inability of the fitted mixture model to provide a reasonable partition of the data. It is possible to show that the ICL criterion is essentially the ordinary BIC penalized by the substraction of the estimated mean entropy, which is a measure of inability—see Biernacki et al. (2000) and McLachlan and Peel (2000, pp. 216) for details. When choosing between the FM-SN and the FM-ST models with two components, our simulation results for the PS case have shown that this measure is often larger for the FM-ST model.

4.5 Application with Real Data

As an application of the methodology proposed in this work, we consider the body mass index for men aged between 18 and 80 years. The data set comes from the National Health and Nutrition Examination Survey, made by the National Center for Health Statistics (NCHS) of the Center for Disease Control (CDC) in the USA. The problem of obesity has attracted attention in the last few years due to its strong relationship with many chronic diseases. Body mass index (BMI, kg/m^2) has become the standard measure for overweight and obesity. BMI is defined as the ratio of body weight in kilograms and body height in meters squared.

This data set was analyzed by Lin et al. (2007a), who considered the reports made in 1999–2000 and 2001–2002. Originally, the set had 4579 participants with BMI records. However, to explore the pattern of mixture, they considered only those participants who have their weights within [39.50 kg, 70.00 kg] and [95.01 kg, 196.80 kg]. The remaining data set consists of 1069 participants in the first subgroup and 1054 in the second subgroup. The models FM-NOR, FM-T, FM-SN, and FM-ST, always with two components, were fitted by Lin et al. (2007a). In this paper, we revisit the BMI data with the aim of providing additional insight by using FM-SMSN models.

Table 4.5 contains the maximum likelihood estimates (MLE) of the parameters of the five models: FM-NOR, FM-SN, FM-ST, FM-SCN, and FM-SSL, besides their corresponding standard errors (SE), computed via the information-based method presented in Sect. 4.3. For model comparison, we also computed the AIC, BIC, EDC, and ICL criteria. The criteria values, except ICL, indicate that the FM-SMSN models with heavy tails (FM-ST, FM-SCN, and FM-SSL) have a significantly better fit than the FM-NOR and FM-SN models. According to these criteria, contrary to Lin et al. (2007a), the FM-SSL model has the best fitting result. In Fig. 4.4, we plot the profile log-likelihood of the parameter ν for the FM-SSL and FM-ST models. It shows once again that the FM-SN model is not favorable for this data set since, in both cases, the profile log-likelihood has a significant drop for small values of ν.

Now we compare the FM-NOR, FM-SSL, and FM-ST models when they are applied to density estimation. We display the fitting results superimposed on a single set of coordinate axes in Fig. 4.5. Based on the graphical visualization, it appears that the FM-SSL and the FM-ST models have quite reasonable and better fit than

Table 4.5 Maximum likelihood estimation results for fitting various mixture models to the BMI data

Parameter	FM-NOR		FM-SN		FM-ST		FM-SCN		FM-SSL	
	MLE	SE	MLE	SE	MLE	SE	MLE	SE	MLE	SE
p_1	0.391	0.0188	0.528	0.0125	0.538	0.0142	0.538	0.0140	0.536	0.0135
μ_1	21.412	0.0936	19.500	0.2429	19.572	0.2432	19.487	0.2363	19.512	0.2372
μ_2	32.548	0.3681	28.760	0.1456	29.100	0.1652	29.023	0.1651	28.972	0.1544
σ_1^2	4.071	0.0873	14.365	0.2841	12.916	0.3072	12.864	0.3022	9.896	0.2636
σ_2^2	41.191	0.1578	63.217	0.1580	45.841	0.3100	44.543	0.4440	36.115	0.3414
λ_1	–	–	1.902	0.3446	1.900	0.3723	2.003	0.3973	1.955	0.3636
λ_2	–	–	10.588	2.7408	7.131	1.8474	7.656	2.1135	8.330	2.1402
ν	–	–	–	–	8.759	2.1238	0.141	0.061	2.421	0.4169
γ	–	–	–	–	–	–	0.284	0.069	–	–
Log-lik	−6911.76		−6868.59		−6855.34		−6854.37		−6855.28	
AIC	13,833.35		13,750.89		13,726.67		13,726.73		13,726.56	
BIC	13,961.61		13,790.46		13,771.89		13,777.61		13,771.78	
EDC	13,869.25		13,801.44		13,784.12		13,791.36		13,784.00	
ICL	14,280.49		13,865.16		13,898.14		13,902.63		13,884.41	

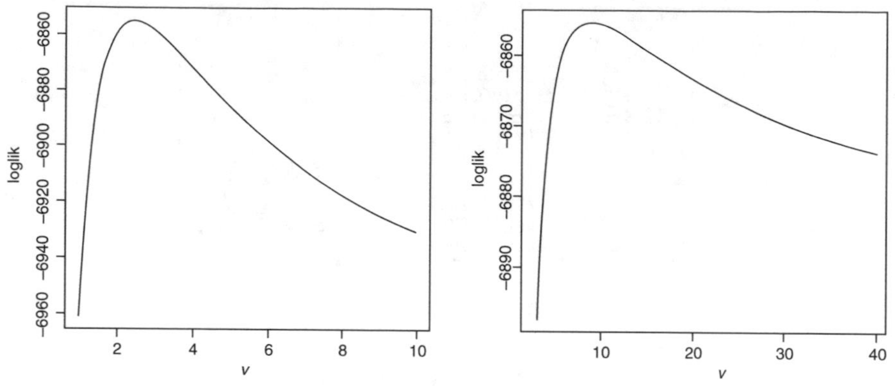

Fig. 4.4 Plot of the profile log-likelihood of the parameter ν for fitting the BMI data with a two component. Left: FM-SSL model; right: FM-ST model

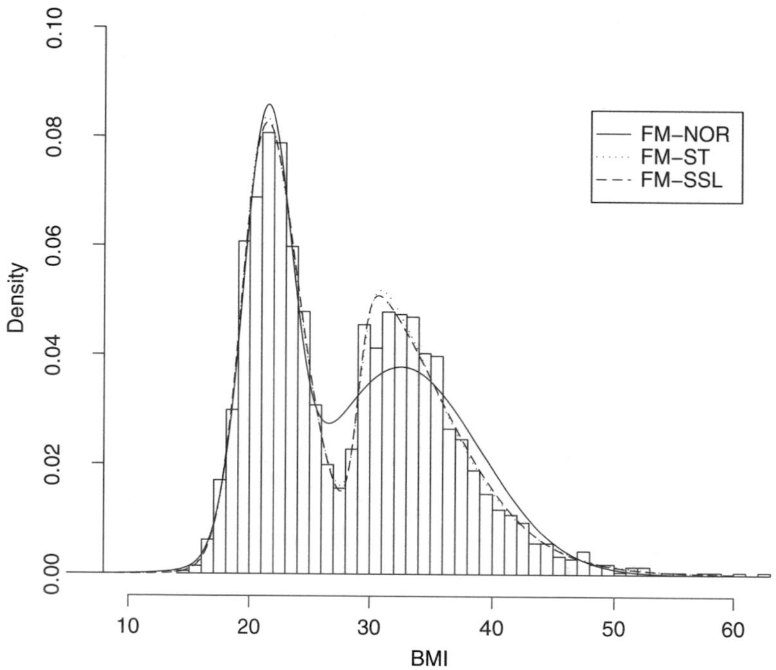

Fig. 4.5 Histogram of BMI data with fitted FM-NOR, FM-ST, and FM-SSL models with two components

the FM-NOR model. It is also important to emphasize that the fitted FM-ST and FM-SSL densities practically coincide. This is the case also with the log-likelihood values (log-lik) given in Table 4.5.

Chapter 5
Multivariate Mixture Modeling Using SMSN Distributions

In this chapter we consider a flexible class of models, with elements that are finite mixtures of multivariate scale mixtures of skew-normal distributions. A general EM-type algorithm is employed for iteratively computing parameter estimates and this is discussed with emphasis on finite mixtures of skew-normal, skew-t, skew-slash, and skew-contaminated normal distributions. Further, a general information-based method for approximating the asymptotic covariance matrix of the estimates is also presented. This part of the theory is based on Cabral et al. (2012), extending results of Lin (2009) and 2010. The proposed EM-type algorithm and methods are implemented in the R package `mixsmsn` (Prates et al. 2013). For a comprehensive survey on alternative definitions of skew-t and skew-normal distributions and its applications in the context of mixture models, we refer to Lee and McLachlan (2013, 2014, 2016), and Lin et al. (2018).

5.1 Introduction

For continuous multivariate data, both in the applied and methodological contexts, much attention has been focussed on the use of normal or Student-t mixture components, hereafter FM-NOR and FM-T models, respectively. They can be easily fitted iteratively by parameter estimation via the expectation maximization (EM) algorithm of Dempster et al. (1977); see also McLachlan and Krishnan (2008). The FM-T model has an extra attractiveness because the Student-t distribution involves an additional tuning parameter (the degrees of freedom) which is useful for outlier accommodation. Developments about the FM-T model include McLachlan and Peel (2000), Shoham (2002), Shoham et al. (2003), Lin et al. (2004), Wang et al. (2004), Yu et al. (2006), and Sfikas et al. (2007).

Although these models are attractive, there is a need to check the distributional assumptions of the mixture components, because the data can present skewness

V. H. Lachos Dávila et al., *Finite Mixture of Skewed Distributions*,
SpringerBriefs in Statistics, https://doi.org/10.1007/978-3-319-98029-4_5

or heavy-tailed behavior. As an alternative to univariate symmetrical mixtures, Lin et al. (2007b) proposed a mixture framework based on the skew-normal (SN) distribution (Azzalini 1985), in order to efficiently deal with population heterogeneity and skewness. This work was extended by Lin et al. (2007a), where they also considered robustness to discrepant observations, using mixtures of the Student-t skewed (ST) distributions defined in Azzalini and Capitanio (2003). Statistical mixture modeling based on normal, Student-t, and SN distributions can be viewed as a special case of the ST mixture modeling. See also Cabral et al. (2008) for an alternative point of view using a Bayesian approach.

Basso et al. (2010) considered estimation for univariate finite mixtures where components are members of the flexible class of scale mixtures of skew-normal distributions (SMSN) (Lachos et al. 2010), which is a subclass of the skew-elliptical class proposed by Branco and Dey (2001). As commented in Chap. 2, this subclass contains the entire family of normal independent distributions (Lange and Sinsheimer 1993).

Lin (2009) has proposed multivariate SN mixture models, and Pyne et al. (2009) and Lin (2010) have proposed multivariate ST mixture models, using the skew elliptical class introduced by Sahu et al. (2003). In this chapter we present mixture models where components are members of the SMSN class, as proposed in Cabral et al. (2012) and Prates et al. (2013). The multivariate SMSN distributions used are developed primarily from the multivariate SN distribution proposed in Azzalini and Dalla-Valle (1996). In contrast with previous developments, the version used here allows us to develop a very simple EM-type algorithm, eliminating some difficulties like Monte Carlo integration when dealing with SN, ST, or SCN components, which has as a consequence a considerably reduction of the computational time. Moreover, our proposal extends (Basso et al. 2010) and the Lin's papers also, in the sense that, by definition, the SMSN class contains as proper elements univariate and multivariate versions of some known scale mixtures of the SN distributions.

The main advances introduced here are: (1) a unified framework for maximum likelihood estimation through an EM-type algorithm with closed form expressions for the E-step in most of the cases considered; (2) a unified methodology to approximate the asymptotic covariance matrix of estimates; (3) an extensive simulation study of properties of the estimates, including consistency, model fit analysis and ability in clustering observations; (4) A R package `mixsmsn` (Prates et al. 2013), available on CRAN, where the proposed methods have been implemented.

The remainder of this chapter is organized as follows. In Sect. 5.2 we propose the finite mixture of SMSN distributions (FM-SMSN) and the corresponding EM-type algorithm. Further, some comments about the existence of the maximum likelihood estimator for FM-SMSN models are given. The related observed information matrix is derived analytically in Sect. 5.3. The methodology proposed for the FM-SMSN models is illustrated in Sect. 5.4, where we proceed a simulation study and an analysis of a real data set. In these examples, besides model fit, we focus on the clustering of observations, since currently most of the existing model-based cluster analysis are based on normal or Student-t mixtures. We show that the FM-SMSN is a relevant alternative to these families, giving practitioners a more flexible choice when estimating the cluster structure for their data at hand.

5.2 The Proposed Model

In this section, we define the *multivariate finite mixture of SMSN distributions (FM-SMSN model)*. Consider a set of independent data vectors $\mathbf{Y}_i$, for $i = 1, \ldots, n$, taken from a G-component mixture of SMSN densities given as

$$f(\mathbf{y}|\boldsymbol{\theta}) = \sum_{j=1}^{G} p_j g(\mathbf{y}|\boldsymbol{\mu}_j, \boldsymbol{\Sigma}_j, \boldsymbol{\lambda}_j, \boldsymbol{\nu}_j), \quad p_j \geq 0, \sum_{j=1}^{G} p_j = 1, \tag{5.1}$$

where $\boldsymbol{\theta} = ((\boldsymbol{\theta}_1^\top, p_1), \ldots, (\boldsymbol{\theta}_g^\top, p_G))^\top$, with $\boldsymbol{\theta}_j = (\boldsymbol{\mu}_j^\top, \boldsymbol{\alpha}_j^\top, \boldsymbol{\lambda}_j^\top, \boldsymbol{\nu}_j^\top)^\top$, $j = 1, \ldots, G$, being the component specific vector of parameters, $g(\cdot|\boldsymbol{\theta}_j)$ is the $\text{SMSN}_p(\boldsymbol{\theta}_j)$ density and p_j's are the mixing probabilities. Recalling that $\boldsymbol{\alpha}_j$ denotes a vector with the elements of the upper triangular matrix of $\boldsymbol{\Sigma}_j$. We assume that the distributions of the mixing scale factors are identical to $H(\cdot; \boldsymbol{\nu})$ and thus $\boldsymbol{\theta}_j = (\boldsymbol{\mu}_j^\top, \boldsymbol{\alpha}_j^\top, \boldsymbol{\lambda}_j^\top, \boldsymbol{\nu}^\top)^\top$, for $j = 1, \ldots, G$.

As usual in the EM framework for mixtures (McLachlan and Peel 2000, Sec 2.8.2), we introduce a set of latent component indicators $\mathbf{Z}_i = (Z_{i1}, \ldots, Z_{iG})^\top$, $i = 1, \ldots, n$, where the coordinate j is a binary random variable defined as

$$Z_{ij} = \begin{cases} 1, & \text{if } \mathbf{Y}_i \text{ belongs to group } j, \\ 0, & \text{otherwise} \end{cases} \tag{5.2}$$

and $\sum_{j=1}^{G} Z_{ij} = 1$. That is,

$$\mathbf{Y}_i|Z_{ij} = 1 \sim \text{SMSN}_p(\boldsymbol{\mu}_j, \boldsymbol{\Sigma}_j, \boldsymbol{\lambda}_j, \boldsymbol{\nu}). \tag{5.3}$$

The indicators $\mathbf{Z}_1, \ldots, \mathbf{Z}_n$ are independent, each one with multinomial distribution, i.e., $\mathbf{Z}_i \sim \text{Multinomial}(1; p_1 \ldots, p_G)$.

From (5.3) along with (3.18)–(3.20), it follows that the hierarchical representation for the FM-SMSN model can be written as

$$\begin{aligned} \mathbf{Y}_i|U_i = u_i, T_i = t_i, Z_{ij} = 1 &\sim \text{N}_p(\boldsymbol{\mu}_j + \boldsymbol{\Delta}_j t_i, u_i^{-1}\boldsymbol{\Gamma}_j), \\ T_i|U_i = u_i, Z_{ij} = 1 &\sim \text{HN}(0, u_i^{-1}), \\ U_i|Z_{ij} = 1 &\sim H(u_i|\boldsymbol{\nu}), \\ \mathbf{Z}_i &\sim \text{Multinomial}(1; p_1 \ldots, p_g), \end{aligned} \tag{5.4}$$

$i = 1, \ldots, n, \;\; j = 1, \ldots, G$, where

$$\boldsymbol{\Delta}_j = \boldsymbol{\Sigma}_j^{1/2}\boldsymbol{\delta}_j, \ \boldsymbol{\delta}_j = \frac{\boldsymbol{\lambda}_j}{\sqrt{1+\boldsymbol{\lambda}_j^\top\boldsymbol{\lambda}_j}}, \quad \boldsymbol{\Gamma}_j = \boldsymbol{\Sigma}_j - \boldsymbol{\Delta}_j\boldsymbol{\Delta}_j^\top.$$

If $U_i = 1$ (that is, the skew-normal case) the model is named FM-SN, if $U_i \sim$ Gamma$(\nu/2, \nu/2)$ (the skew-t case) it is named FM-ST and so on.

5.2.1 *Maximum Likelihood Estimation via EM Algorithm*

In this subsection, we implement the EM-type algorithm for the estimation of the parameters of the FM-SMSN model. Before we start, let us make some comments about the existence of the maximum likelihood estimator for finite mixture models.

It is well known that the likelihood associated with the FM-NOR model may be unbounded—see Frühwirth-Schnatter (2006, Chapter 6), for example. FM-SMSN models also have this feature: for instance, let $\mathbf{y}_i$, $i = 1, \ldots, n$, be a random sample from a mixture of two SMSN densities, $\mathrm{SMSN}_q(\cdot|\boldsymbol{\mu}, \boldsymbol{\Sigma}_1, \boldsymbol{\lambda}_1, \boldsymbol{\nu})$ with weight $p \in (0, 1)$ and $\mathrm{SMSN}_q(\cdot|\boldsymbol{\mu}, \boldsymbol{\Sigma}_2, \boldsymbol{\lambda}_2, \boldsymbol{\nu})$. Fixing p, $\boldsymbol{\Sigma}_1$, $\boldsymbol{\lambda}_1$, $\boldsymbol{\lambda}_2$, and $\boldsymbol{\nu}$, we have that the likelihood function $L(\cdot)$ evaluated at $\boldsymbol{\mu} = \mathbf{y}_1$ satisfies

$$L(\mathbf{y}_1, \boldsymbol{\Sigma}_2) = g(\boldsymbol{\Sigma}_2)\prod_{i=2}^{n}(c_i + h_i(\boldsymbol{\Sigma}_2)) > g(\boldsymbol{\Sigma}_2)\prod_{i=2}^{n} c_i,$$

where

$$g(\boldsymbol{\Sigma}_2) = \left(p(2\pi)^{-q/2}|\boldsymbol{\Sigma}_1|^{-1/2} + (1-p)(2\pi)^{-q/2}|\boldsymbol{\Sigma}_2|^{-1/2}\right)\int_0^\infty \kappa(u)^{-q/2}dH(u),$$

$$c_i = p\mathrm{SMSN}_q(\mathbf{y}_i|\mathbf{y}_1, \boldsymbol{\Sigma}_1, \boldsymbol{\lambda}_1, \boldsymbol{\nu}),$$

$$h_i(\boldsymbol{\Sigma}_2) = (1-p)\mathrm{SMSN}_q(\mathbf{y}_i|\mathbf{y}_1, \boldsymbol{\Sigma}_2, \boldsymbol{\lambda}_2, \boldsymbol{\nu}), \qquad i = 2, \ldots, n$$

and $|\cdot|$ denotes the determinant of a matrix—the inequality is valid because c_i and $h_i(\boldsymbol{\Sigma}_2)$ are positive. Now, we can choose a sequence of positive definite matrixes $(\boldsymbol{\Sigma}_2^{(m)})$, $m \in \mathbb{N}$, such that $\lim_{m\to\infty} |\boldsymbol{\Sigma}_2^{(m)}| = 0$. Then, because $\prod_{i=2}^n c_i > 0$ and $\lim_{m\to\infty} g(\boldsymbol{\Sigma}_2^{(m)}) = +\infty$, we have that $\lim_{m\to\infty} L(y_1, \boldsymbol{\Sigma}_2^{(m)}) = +\infty$.

Thus, our choice is to follow Nityasuddhi and Böhning (2003). Quoting them: "it is only fair not to speak about maximum-likelihood estimates, but rather about the estimates which the EM algorithm provides (some sort of solution of the score equation) and call them EM algorithm estimates."

Having done these remarks, let us present the algorithm. We have that, from representation (5.4), the complete log-likelihood function is

$$\ell_c(\boldsymbol{\theta}|\mathbf{y},\mathbf{t},\mathbf{u},\mathbf{z}) = c + \sum_{i=1}^{n}\sum_{j=1}^{G} Z_{ij}\Big[\log(p_j) - \frac{1}{2}\log|\boldsymbol{\Gamma}_j| - \frac{u_i}{2}(\mathbf{y}_i - \boldsymbol{\mu}_j - \boldsymbol{\Delta}_j t_i)^\top \boldsymbol{\Gamma}_j^{-1}(\mathbf{y}_i - \boldsymbol{\mu}_j - \boldsymbol{\Delta}_j t_i) + \log(h(u_i;\boldsymbol{\nu}))\Big],$$

where c is a constant and $\mathbf{z} = (\mathbf{z}_1^\top, \ldots, \mathbf{z}_n^\top)^\top$. The conditional expectations involved in the E-step, that is, the computation of $Q(\boldsymbol{\theta}|\widehat{\boldsymbol{\theta}}^{(k)}) = E[\ell_c(\boldsymbol{\theta}|\mathbf{y},\mathbf{t},\mathbf{u},\mathbf{z})|\mathbf{y},\widehat{\boldsymbol{\theta}}^{(k)}]$, are

$$\widehat{z}_{ij}^{(k)} = E[Z_{ij}|\mathbf{y}_i,\widehat{\boldsymbol{\theta}}^{(k)}],\quad \widehat{zu}_{ij}^{(k)} = E[Z_{ij}U_i|\mathbf{y}_i,\widehat{\boldsymbol{\theta}}^{(k)}],\quad \widehat{zut}_{ij}^{(k)} = E[Z_{ij}U_iT_i|\mathbf{y}_i,\widehat{\boldsymbol{\theta}}^{(k)}],$$

$$\text{and}\quad \widehat{zut^2}_{ij}^{(k)} = E[Z_{ij}U_iT_i^2|\mathbf{y}_i,\widehat{\boldsymbol{\theta}}^{(k)}].$$

The expression for $\widehat{zu}_{ij}^{(k)}$ can be obtained using the relation

$$E[Z_{ij}U_i|\mathbf{Y}_i] = E[Z_{ij}E[U_i|\mathbf{Y}_i, Z_{ij}]|\mathbf{Y}_i].$$

For each fixed $\mathbf{y}_i$, the distribution of $q(\mathbf{Y}_i, Z_{ij}) = Z_{ij}E[U_i|\mathbf{Y}_i, Z_{ij}]$ given $\mathbf{Y}_i = \mathbf{y}_i$ is binary, assuming the value $q(\mathbf{y}_i, 1) = E[U_i|\mathbf{Y}_i = \mathbf{y}_i, Z_{ij} = 1]$ with probability $P(Z_{ij} = 1|\mathbf{Y}_i = \mathbf{y}_i) = \widehat{z}_{ij}^{(k)}$ and zero with probability $P(Z_{ij} = 0|\mathbf{Y}_i = \mathbf{y}_i)$. It is straightforward to show that

$$\widehat{z}_{ij}^{(k)} = \frac{\widehat{p}_j^{(k)} g(\mathbf{y}_i|\widehat{\boldsymbol{\theta}}_j^{(k)})}{\sum_{j=1}^{G}\widehat{p}_j^{(k)} g(\mathbf{y}_i|\widehat{\boldsymbol{\theta}}_j^{(k)})} \tag{5.5}$$

and that the distribution of $U_i|\mathbf{Y}_i = \mathbf{y}_i, Z_{ij} = 1$ is the distribution of $U_i|\mathbf{Y}_0 = \mathbf{y}_i$ when $\mathbf{Y}_0 \sim \text{SMSN}(\widehat{\boldsymbol{\theta}}_j^{(k)})$. Using similar arguments in order to obtain the other conditional expectations, we have

$$\widehat{zu}_{ij}^{(k)} = \widehat{z}_{ij}^{(k)}\widehat{u}_{ij}^{(k)},\quad \widehat{zut}_{ij}^{(k)} = \widehat{z}_{ij}^{(k)}\widehat{ut}_{ij}^{(k)}\quad\text{and}\quad \widehat{zut^2}_{ij}^{(k)} = \widehat{z}_{ij}^{(k)}\widehat{ut^2}_{ij}^{(k)}. \tag{5.6}$$

These expressions can be evaluated using their counterparts for the one-component case, given in Sect. 3.3.1.

We have adopted the same strategy, used in Chap. 3, to obtain $\widehat{\boldsymbol{\nu}}^{(k+1)}$, by direct maximization of the actual marginal log-likelihood (ECME algorithm), avoiding then the process of computing $E[Z_{ij}\log(h(u_i;\boldsymbol{\nu}))|\mathbf{y}_i,\widehat{\boldsymbol{\theta}}]$. It can be summarized as follows:

E-step: Given $\boldsymbol{\theta} = \boldsymbol{\theta}^{(k)}$, compute $\widehat{z}_{ij}^{(k)}$, $\widehat{zu}_{ij}^{(k)}$, $\widehat{zut}_{ij}^{(k)}$ and $\widehat{zut^2}_{ij}^{(k)}$, for $i = 1, \ldots, n$ and $j = 1, \ldots, G$.

M-step:

1. For $j = 1, \ldots, G$, update $\widehat{p}_j^{(k)}$, $\widehat{\boldsymbol{\mu}}_j^{(k)}$, $\widehat{\boldsymbol{\Gamma}}_j^{(k)}$ and $\widehat{\boldsymbol{\Delta}}_j^{(k)}$ using the following closed form expressions

$$\widehat{p}_j^{(k+1)} = n^{-1}\sum_{i=1}^{n}\widehat{z}_{ij}^{(k)};$$

$$\widehat{\boldsymbol{\mu}}_j^{(k+1)} = \sum_{i=1}^{n}(\widehat{zu}_{ij}^{(k)}\mathbf{y}_i - \widehat{zut}_{ij}^{(k)}\boldsymbol{\Delta}_j^{(k)})/\sum_{i=1}^{n}\widehat{zu}_{ij}^{(k)};$$

$$\widehat{\boldsymbol{\Delta}}_j^{(k+1)} = \left[\sum_{i=1}^{n}\widehat{zut}_{ij}^{(k)}(\mathbf{y}_i - \widehat{\boldsymbol{\mu}}_j^{(k+1)})\right]/\sum_{i=1}^{n}\widehat{zut^2}_{ij}^{(k)};$$

$$\begin{aligned}\widehat{\boldsymbol{\Gamma}}_j^{(k+1)} = \left(\sum_{i=1}^{n}\widehat{z}_{ij}^{(k)}\right)^{-1}\sum_{i=1}^{n}\Big(&\widehat{zu}_{ij}^{(k)}(\mathbf{y}_i - \widehat{\boldsymbol{\mu}}_j^{(k+1)})(\mathbf{y}_i - \widehat{\boldsymbol{\mu}}_j^{(k+1)})^\top \\ &-\left[(\mathbf{y}_i - \widehat{\boldsymbol{\mu}}_j^{(k+1)})(\widehat{\boldsymbol{\Delta}}_j^{(k+1)})^\top + \widehat{\boldsymbol{\Delta}}_j^{(k+1)}(\mathbf{y}_i - \widehat{\boldsymbol{\mu}}_j^{(k+1)})^\top\right]\widehat{zut}_{ij}^{(k)} \\ &+\widehat{\boldsymbol{\Delta}}_j^{(k+1)}(\widehat{\boldsymbol{\Delta}}_j^{(k+1)})^\top\widehat{zut^2}_{ij}^{(k)}\Big);\end{aligned}$$

2. Update $\boldsymbol{\nu}^{(k)}$ by maximizing the actual marginal log-likelihood function, obtaining

$$\widehat{\boldsymbol{\nu}}^{(k+1)} = \arg\max_{\boldsymbol{\nu}}\sum_{i=1}^{n}\log\left(\sum_{j=1}^{G}p_j g\left(\mathbf{y}_i|\widehat{\boldsymbol{\mu}}_j^{(k+1)}, \widehat{\boldsymbol{\Sigma}}_j^{(k+1)}, \widehat{\boldsymbol{\lambda}}_j^{(k+1)}, \boldsymbol{\nu}\right)\right).$$

A more parsimonious model is achieved by supposing $\boldsymbol{\Gamma}_1 = \ldots = \boldsymbol{\Gamma}_g = \boldsymbol{\Gamma}$, which can be seen as an extension of the FM-NOR model with restricted variance–covariance components. In this case, the updates for $\widehat{p}_j^{(k)}$, $\widehat{\boldsymbol{\mu}}_j^{(k)}$, and $\widehat{\boldsymbol{\Delta}}_j^{(k)}$ remain the same, and the update for $\widehat{\boldsymbol{\Gamma}}^{(k)}$ is given as

$$\widehat{\boldsymbol{\Gamma}}^{(k+1)} = \frac{1}{n}\sum_{i=1}^{n}\sum_{j=1}^{G}\widehat{z}_{ij}^{(k)}\widehat{\boldsymbol{\Gamma}}_j^{(k+1)}.$$

The iterations are repeated until a suitable convergence rule is satisfied, e.g., if $||\boldsymbol{\theta}^{(k+1)} - \boldsymbol{\theta}^{(k)}||$ is sufficiently small or until some distance involving two successive evaluations of the actual log-likelihood $\ell(\boldsymbol{\theta})$, like $||\ell(\boldsymbol{\theta}^{(k+1)}) - \ell(\boldsymbol{\theta}^{(k)})||$ or $||\ell(\boldsymbol{\theta}^{(k+1)})/\ell(\boldsymbol{\theta}^{(k)}) - 1||$, is small enough. See Dias and Wedel (2004) for a discussion in the context of mixtures of univariate normal distributions.

For some distributions, like SN, ST, and SCN, we can see from the results above that the updating expressions for the location, scale, and skewness parameters are written in a closed form. But the same is not true when dealing with finite mixtures of the skew-t defined by Lin (2010). In this sense, our work differs from Lin's works, where in the E-step Monte Carlo integration is used (see eq. 22 in Lin 2010) or the moments or the truncated multinormal distribution are computed (see Theorem 1 in Lin 2009). Thus, our models and algorithms deal with these issues in a more friendly way, implying in a substantial computing time reduction.

In a related recent paper, Karlis and Santourian (2009) proposed to fit skewed heavy-tailed components using finite mixtures of normal inverse Gaussian (NIG) components. They argue that an advantage of this approach when comparing with Lin's works is the lower computational cost, being the most complicated part of the evaluation of the Bessel function, which is easily available in statistical packages. This property is also shared by the FM-SMSN models considered here, because all we need is to evaluate, in the E-step, the normal and the Student-t distributions functions. In the SSL case, the evaluation of some integrals through the routine `integrate` is also required.

5.3 The Observed Information Matrix

We again use the alternative method suggested by Basford et al. (1997), which consists in approximating the inverse of the asymptotic covariance matrix of $\widehat{\boldsymbol{\theta}}$ by $\mathbf{J}_o(\widehat{\boldsymbol{\theta}}|\mathbf{Y}_j)$, where

$$\mathbf{J}_o(\boldsymbol{\theta}|\mathbf{Y}_j) = \sum_{i=1}^{n} \mathbf{s}_i \mathbf{s}_i^\top, \quad \text{with} \quad \mathbf{s}_i = \frac{\partial}{\partial \boldsymbol{\theta}} \log f(\mathbf{y}_i|\boldsymbol{\theta}), \tag{5.7}$$

where $f(\cdot|\boldsymbol{\theta})$ is the FM-SMSN density in (5.1) (with $\boldsymbol{\nu}_1 = \ldots = \boldsymbol{\nu}_g = \boldsymbol{\nu}$). That is, $\mathbf{s}_i$ is the score vector associated with $\mathbf{y}_i$. To simplify the notation, let us define

$$\mathrm{S}_j(\mathbf{y}_i) = g(\mathbf{y}_i|\boldsymbol{\theta}_j), \quad s_{i,\mu_r} = \frac{\partial}{\partial \boldsymbol{\mu}_r} \log f(\mathbf{y}_i|\boldsymbol{\theta}) \quad \text{and} \quad D_{\mu_r}(\mathrm{S}_r(\mathbf{y}_i)) = \frac{\partial \mathrm{S}_r(\mathbf{y}_i)}{\partial \boldsymbol{\mu}_r}.$$

Partial derivatives with respect to the other component specific parameters are denoted in an analogous way. Then, we have

$$s_{i,p_r} = \frac{\mathrm{S}_r(\mathbf{y}_i) - \mathrm{S}_g(\mathbf{y}_i)}{f(\mathbf{y}_i|\boldsymbol{\theta})}, \quad i = 1, \ldots, n, \; r = 1, \ldots, G-1,$$

$$s_{i,\mu_r} = \frac{p_r D_{\mu_r}(\mathrm{S}_r(\mathbf{y}_i))}{f(\mathbf{y}_i|\boldsymbol{\theta})}, \quad s_{i,\alpha_{rk}} = \frac{p_r D_{\alpha_{rk}}(\mathrm{S}_r(\mathbf{y}_i))}{f(\mathbf{y}_i|\boldsymbol{\theta})},$$

$$s_{i,\boldsymbol{\lambda}_r} = \frac{p_r D_{\boldsymbol{\lambda}_r}(\mathrm{S}_r(\mathbf{y}_i))}{f(\mathbf{y}_i|\boldsymbol{\theta})}, \quad s_{i,\boldsymbol{\nu}} = \frac{\sum_{j=1}^{G} p_j D_{\boldsymbol{\nu}}(\mathrm{S}_j(\mathbf{y}_i))}{f(\mathbf{y}_i|\boldsymbol{\theta})},$$
$$i = 1, \ldots, n, \; r = 1, \ldots, G,$$

where $\boldsymbol{\alpha}_{rk}$ denotes the kth element of $\boldsymbol{\alpha}_r$. Note that $D_{\boldsymbol{\nu}}(\mathrm{S}_j(\mathbf{y}_i))$ must be obtained for each particular case mentioned in Sect. 3.5 (i.e., ST, SSL, and SCN). After some algebraic manipulation and using the notation

$$\mathrm{I}_{ir}^{\Phi}(w) = \int_0^{\infty} u_i^w \exp\left\{-\frac{1}{2}u_i \mathrm{d}_{ir}\right\} \Phi(u_i^{1/2}\mathrm{A}_{ir}) dH(u_i; \boldsymbol{\nu}),$$

$$\mathrm{I}_{ir}^{\phi}(w) = \int_0^{\infty} u_i^w \exp\left\{-\frac{1}{2}u_i \mathrm{d}_{ir}\right\} \phi(u_i^{1/2}\mathrm{A}_{ir}) dH(u_i; \boldsymbol{\nu}),$$

where $\mathrm{d}_{ir} = \mathrm{d}_{\boldsymbol{\Sigma}_r}(\mathbf{y}_i, \boldsymbol{\mu}_r)$ and $\mathrm{A}_{ir} = \boldsymbol{\lambda}_r^{\top}\boldsymbol{\Sigma}_r^{-1/2}(\mathbf{y}_i - \boldsymbol{\mu}_r)$, one can show that

$$D_{\boldsymbol{\mu}_r}(\mathrm{S}_r(\mathbf{y}_i)) = \frac{2|\boldsymbol{\Sigma}_r|^{-1/2}}{(2\pi)^{p/2}}\left[\left(\frac{\partial \mathrm{A}_{ir}}{\partial \boldsymbol{\mu}_r}\right)\mathrm{I}_{ir}^{\phi}\left(\frac{p+1}{2}\right) - \frac{1}{2}\left(\frac{\partial \mathrm{d}_{ir}}{\partial \boldsymbol{\mu}_r}\right)\mathrm{I}_{ir}^{\Phi}\left(\frac{p}{2}+1\right)\right],$$

$$D_{\boldsymbol{\alpha}_{rk}}(\mathrm{S}_r(\mathbf{y}_i)) = \frac{2}{(2\pi)^{p/2}}\left[\left(\frac{\partial|\boldsymbol{\Sigma}_r|^{-1/2}}{\partial \boldsymbol{\alpha}_{rk}}\right)\mathrm{I}_{ir}^{\Phi}\left(\frac{p}{2}\right) - \frac{1}{2}\left(\frac{\partial \mathrm{d}_{ir}}{\partial \boldsymbol{\alpha}_{rk}}\right)|\boldsymbol{\Sigma}_r|^{-1/2}\mathrm{I}_{ir}^{\Phi}\left(\frac{p}{2}+1\right)\right.$$
$$\left. + |\boldsymbol{\Sigma}_r|^{-1/2}\left(\frac{\partial \mathrm{A}_{ir}}{\partial \boldsymbol{\alpha}_{rk}}\right)\mathrm{I}_{ir}^{\phi}\left(\frac{p+1}{2}\right)\right],$$

$$D_{\boldsymbol{\lambda}_r}(\mathrm{S}_r(\mathbf{y}_i)) = \frac{2|\boldsymbol{\Sigma}_r|^{-1/2}}{(2\pi)^{p/2}}\left(\frac{\partial \mathrm{A}_{ir}}{\partial \boldsymbol{\lambda}_r}\right)\mathrm{I}_{ir}^{\phi}\left(\frac{p+1}{2}\right).$$

Expressions for the derivatives are standard and are not given here. Direct substitution of $H(\cdot; \boldsymbol{\nu})$ in the integrals above yields the following results for each distribution considered in this work, namely

5.3.1 The Skew-Normal Distribution

$$\mathrm{I}_{ir}^{\Phi}(w) = \exp\{-\mathrm{d}_{ir}/2\}\Phi(\mathrm{A}_{ir}), \quad \mathrm{I}_{ir}^{\phi}(w) = \exp\{-\mathrm{d}_{ir}/2\}\phi(\mathrm{A}_{ir}).$$

5.3.2 *The Skew-t Distribution*

$$I_{ir}^{\Phi}(w) = \frac{2^w \nu^{\nu/2}\Gamma(w+\nu/2)}{\sqrt{2\pi}\Gamma(\nu/2)(\nu+d_{ir})^{\nu/2+w}} T\left(\frac{\mathbf{A}_{ir}}{(d_{ir}+\nu)^{1/2}}\sqrt{2w+\nu}|2w+\nu\right),$$

$$I_{ir}^{\phi}(w) = \frac{2^w \nu^{\nu/2}}{\sqrt{2\pi}\Gamma(\nu/2)}\left(\frac{1}{d_{ir}+\mathbf{A}_{ir}^2+\nu}\right)^{\frac{\nu+2w}{2}}\Gamma\left(\frac{\nu+2w}{2}\right),$$

$$D_\nu(S_j(\mathbf{y}_i)) = (2\pi)^{-p/2}|\mathbf{\Sigma}_j|^{-1/2}\Big(I_{ij}^{\Phi}(p/2)(1+\log(\nu/2)-\psi(\nu/2)) - I_{ij}^{\Phi}(1+p/2)$$
$$+\int_0^\infty u_i^{p/2}\log(u_i)\exp\{-u_i d_{ij}/2\}\times\Phi(u_i^{1/2}\mathbf{A}_{ij})h(u_i|\nu)du_i\Big),$$

where $\psi(\cdot)$ denotes the digamma function and $h(\cdot|\nu)$ is the gamma density with both parameters $\nu/2$.

5.3.3 *The Skew-Slash Distribution*

$$I_{ir}^{\Phi}(w) = \frac{2^{2+\nu}\Gamma(w+\nu)}{d_{ir}^{w+\nu}} P_1(w+\nu, d_{ir}/2)E[\Phi(V_{ir}^{1/2})\mathbf{A}_{ir}],$$

$$I_{ir}^{\phi}(w) = \frac{\nu 2^{w+\nu}\Gamma(w+\nu)}{\sqrt{2\pi}(d_{ir}+\mathbf{A}_{ir}^2)^{w+\nu}} P_1\left(w+\nu, \frac{d_{ir}+\mathbf{A}_{ir}^2}{2}\right),$$

where $V_{ir} \sim TG(w+\nu, d_{ir}/2, (0,1))$ and

$$D_\nu(S_j(\mathbf{y}_i)) = 2(2\pi)^{-p/2}|\mathbf{\Sigma}_j|^{-1/2}\Big\{I_{ij}^{\Phi}(p/2+\nu-1)$$
$$+\nu\int_0^1 u_i^{\frac{p}{2}+\nu-1}\log(u_i)\exp\{-u_i d_{ij}/2\}\Phi(u_i^{1/2}\mathbf{A}_{ij})du_i\Big\}.$$

5.3.4 *The Skew-Contaminated Normal Distribution*

$$I_{ir}^{\Phi}(w) = \sqrt{2\pi}\{\nu_1\nu_2^{w-1/2}\phi(d_{ir}|0,1/\nu_2)\Phi(\nu_2^{1/2}\mathbf{A}_{ir}) + (1-\nu_1)\phi(d_{ir})\Phi(\mathbf{A}_{ir})\},$$

$$I_{ir}^{\phi}(w) = \{\nu_1\nu_2^{w-1/2}\phi(d_{ir}+\mathbf{A}_{ir}^2|0,1/\nu_2) + (1-\nu_1)\phi(d_{ir}+\mathbf{A}_{ir}^2)\},$$

$$D_{\nu_1}(S_j(\mathbf{y}_i)) = 2\{\phi_p(y_i|\boldsymbol{\mu}_j,\nu_2^{-1}\mathbf{\Sigma}_j)\Phi(\nu_2^{1/2}\mathbf{A}_{ij}) - \phi_p(y_i|\boldsymbol{\mu}_j,\mathbf{\Sigma}_j)\Phi(\mathbf{A}_{ij})\},$$

$$D_{\nu_2}(S_j(\mathbf{y}_i)) = \nu_1\phi_p(\boldsymbol{\mu}_j,\nu_2^{-1}\mathbf{\Sigma}_j)\{A_{ij}\nu_2^{-1/2}\phi(\nu_2^{1/2}A_{ij}) + \Phi(\nu_2^{1/2}\mathbf{A}_{ij})(p\nu_2^{-1}-d_{ij})\}.$$

In the next section we perform simulation experiments which show evidence that, at least asymptotically, this is a reliable method to provide standard errors estimates in the FM-SNI context. Maybe more accurate estimates could be obtained by using the bootstrap approach (Efron and Tibshirani 1986), but this gain is achieved with the price of an enormous computing time.

5.4 Applications with Simulated and Real Data

In this section we investigate some properties of the SMSN model fit and of the proposed EM-type algorithm by analyzing some artificial and real data sets. The computations were made using the R package `mixsmsn` (Prates et al. 2013), available on CRAN.

5.4.1 Consistency

First, we considered artificial samples generated from a two-component FM-ST model with parameters values $\boldsymbol{\mu}_1 = (2,2)^\top$, $\boldsymbol{\mu}_2 = (-2,-1)^\top$, $p = 0.6$, $\nu = 4$ and

$$\boldsymbol{\lambda}_1 = \boldsymbol{\lambda}_2 = (-5, 10)^\top, \boldsymbol{\Sigma}_1 = \boldsymbol{\Sigma}_2 = \begin{pmatrix} 1.5 & 0 \\ 0 & 1.5 \end{pmatrix}. \tag{5.8}$$

The data sets considered are 500 samples of size $n = 500, 1000, 2000$. Figure 5.1 shows one of these samples ($n = 1000$), with the respective plug-in density contours resulting from fitting the two component FM-ST model. Different colors discriminate the heterogeneous groups. Also, for comparison purposes, the contours of the FM-NOR model fit are presented.

For each data set was fitted the two-component FM-ST model. The following starting values were fixed: $\boldsymbol{\mu}_1 = \boldsymbol{\mu}_2 = \mathbf{0}$, $\boldsymbol{\lambda}_1 = \boldsymbol{\lambda}_2 = (-1, 5)$, $\boldsymbol{\Sigma}_1 = \boldsymbol{\Sigma}_2 = \mathbf{I}_2$,

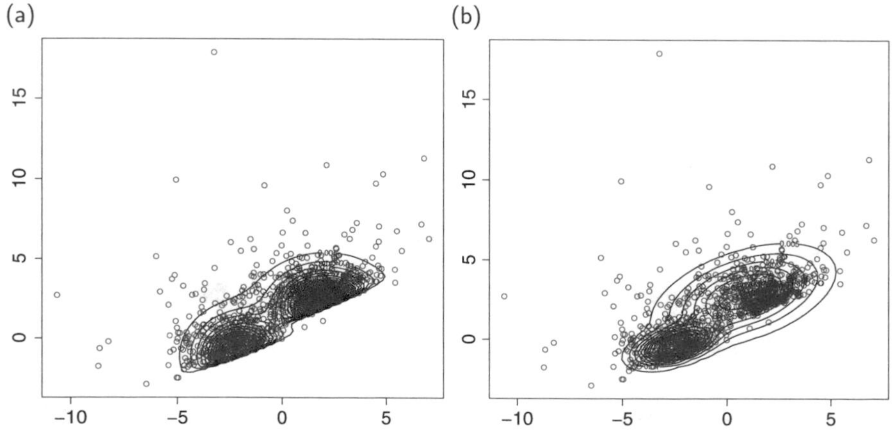

Fig. 5.1 Simulated sample ($n = 1000$) from an FM-ST population and the respective density contours: (**a**) FM-ST fit, (**b**) FM-NOR fit

$\nu = 10$ and $p_1 = 0.5$. We used the convergence rule

$$||\ell(\boldsymbol{\theta}^{(k+1)})/\ell(\boldsymbol{\theta}^{(k)}) - 1|| < 10^{-6}, \tag{5.9}$$

see Sect. 5.2.1. The average values and the corresponding standard deviations of the EM estimates across all samples were computed. Also were computed the average values of the approximate standard deviations of the EM estimates obtained through the information based method described in Sect. 5.3 (IM SD). The results are very satisfactory and are showed in Table 5.1.

We conducted the experiment again, considering now 500 samples generated from a mixture of two SCN distributions with parameters $\boldsymbol{\mu}_1 = (2, 2)^\top$, $\boldsymbol{\mu}_2 = (-4, -3)^\top$, $\boldsymbol{\nu} = (0.4, 0.2)$ and the other parameters as in (5.8). The starting value for $\boldsymbol{\nu}$ is $(0.5, 0.5)$ and, for the remaining parameters, we used the same values of the previous analysis. From these results we can note evidences that the EM estimates have good asymptotic properties.

Results for the FM-SN had a similar pattern than those shown in Tables 5.2 and 5.3, and we omit them. Because of the computationally expensive nature of the procedure in the FM-SSL case, we did not consider it.

5.4.2 *Standard Deviation*

As mention in Sect. 5.3, it is natural to use the inverse of the observed information matrix evaluated at $\widehat{\boldsymbol{\theta}}$ to approximate the asymptotic covariance matrix for EM algorithms. However such calculation is not simple and require enormous algebraical and/or computational effort. We propose to use the method suggested by Basford et al. (1997) to approximate the asymptotic covariance matrix. To study the performance of the proposed method we present a simulation with the following setup:

1. A mixture of two univariate SN distributions. The first component is an $\mathrm{SN}(2, 4, 2)$ distribution with weight 0.2 and the second component is an $\mathrm{SN}(20, 9, -1)$ distribution;
2. A mixture of two univariate ST distributions. The first component is an $\mathrm{ST}(2, 4, 2, 5)$ distribution with weight 0.2 and the second component is an $\mathrm{ST}(20, 9, -1, 5)$ distribution.

For each setup, we generated 1000 samples of size $n = 500, 1000, 2000$ and 5000 and we obtained the average values across all samples in three situations: (1) of the approximate standard deviations of the ML estimates obtained through (5.7) (*gradient method*), (2) of the approximate standard deviations of the ML estimates obtained the inverse of the observed information matrix (*Hessian method*) and (3) of the corresponding standard deviations of the EM estimates across all samples (*SD*). The results are presented in Table 5.3

Table 5.1 Mean and standard deviations (SD) for EM estimates—500 samples from the FM-ST model

		Parameter								
j	Measure	μ_{j1}	μ_{j2}	$\sigma_{j,11}$	$\sigma_{j,12}$	$\sigma_{j,22}$	$\lambda_{j,1}$	$\lambda_{j,2}$	p	ν
$n = 500$										
1	True	(2)	(2)	(1.5)	(0)	(1.5)	(−5)	(10)	(0.6)	(4)
	Mean	2.0089	2.0183	1.5082	0.0191	1.4238	−5.8771	11.4675	0.6011	4.0163
	SD	0.1362	0.0758	0.2501	0.1378	0.1935	8.1513	13.6943	0.0261	0.6372
	IM SD	0.1361	0.0748	0.1044	0.1177	0.0923	8.2137	14.4947	0.0276	0.6454
2	True	(−2)	(−1)	(1.5)	(0)	(1.5)	(−5)	(10)		
	Mean	−2.0062	−0.9906	1.4893	0.0323	1.4684	−7.4445	14.4328		
	SD	0.1696	0.0942	0.2519	0.1914	0.3200	11.4874	18.6441		
	IM SD	0.1656	0.0912	0.1066	0.1607	0.1431	24.5640	41.8629		
$n = 1000$										
1	True	(2)	(2)	(1.5)	(0)	(1.5)	(−5)	(10)	(0.6)	(4)
	Mean	1.9926	2.0075	1.4984	0.0296	1.4442	−4.8715	9.7192	0.6005	3.9975
	SD	0.1057	0.0671	0.2134	0.1480	0.1707	1.3433	2.4639	0.0218	1.2964
	IM SD	0.0965	0.0525	0.0730	0.0823	0.0644	1.3033	2.8196	0.0194	0.4438
2	True	(−2)	(−1)	(1.5)	(0)	(1.5)	(−5)	(10)		
	Mean	−2.0057	−0.9923	1.5046	0.0360	1.4721	−5.2625	10.5147		
	SD	0.1335	0.0683	0.2993	0.3723	0.7048	2.1456	3.9053		
	IM SD	0.1178	0.0649	0.0755	0.1123	0.1019	1.7203	3.5147		
$n = 2000$										
1	True	(2)	(2)	(1.5)	(0)	(1.5)	(−5)	(10)	(0.6)	(4)
	Mean	1.9977	2.0095	1.4857	0.0224	1.4286	−4.7017	9.3066	0.6003	3.8903
	SD	0.0633	0.0344	0.1171	0.0673	0.0979	0.8474	1.6142	0.0135	0.2630
	IM SD	0.0670	0.0369	0.0515	0.0570	0.0446	0.8234	1.7174	0.0137	0.2866
2	True	(−2)	(−1)	(1.5)	(0)	(1.5)	(−5)	(10)		
	Mean	−2.0018	−0.9920	1.4798	0.0251	1.4436	−4.8545	9.6904		
	SD	0.0832	0.0439	0.1265	0.0921	0.1521	1.0636	1.8192		
	IM SD	0.0835	0.0461	0.0529	0.0799	0.0728	0.9680	2.0226		

Table 5.2 Mean and standard deviations (SD) for EM estimates—500 samples from the FM-SCN model

j	Measure	Parameter μ_{j1}	μ_{j2}	$\sigma_{j,11}$	$\sigma_{j,12}$	$\sigma_{j,22}$	$\lambda_{j,1}$	$\lambda_{j,2}$	p	ν_1	ν_2
$n = 500$											
1	True	(2)	(2)	(1.5)	(0)	(1.5)	(−5)	(10)	(0.6)	0.4	0.2
	Mean	1.9890	2.0087	1.4066	0.0263	1.3545	−5.6189	11.3084	0.6004	0.4384	0.1923
	SD	0.1519	0.0838	0.2570	0.1218	0.2047	2.7232	5.4377	0.0239	0.0750	0.0204
	IM SD	0.1501	0.0832	0.1165	0.1035	0.1162	2.4426	5.1227	0.0240	0.0795	0.0338
2	True	(−4)	(−3)	(1.5)	(0)	(1.5)	(−5)	(10)			
	Mean	−3.9961	−2.9772	1.4023	0.0303	1.2993	−6.9303	13.4032			
	SD	0.2013	0.1082	0.2554	0.1601	0.3028	8.6517	16.7808			
	IM SD	0.1914	0.1062	0.1073	0.1384	0.1381	11.4543	23.7004			
$n = 1000$											
1	True	(2)	(2)	(1.5)	(0)	(1.5)	(−5)	(10)	(0.6)	0.4	0.2
	Mean	1.9990	2.0112	1.3988	0.0200	1.3584	−5.0372	10.0564	0.6009	0.4354	0.1913
	SD	0.0974	0.0545	0.1727	0.0791	0.1405	1.2600	2.5854	0.0159	0.0510	0.0154
	IM SD	0.1049	0.0584	0.0805	0.0719	0.0804	1.2677	2.6635	0.0169	0.0545	0.0228
2	True	(−4)	(−3)	(1.5)	(0)	(1.5)	(−5)	(10)			
	Mean	−4.0008	−2.9835	1.3834	0.0274	1.3221	−5.0268	9.9509			
	SD	0.1377	0.0770	0.1737	0.1156	0.2209	1.5273	2.8991			
	IM SD	0.1342	0.0749	0.0736	0.0970	0.0981	1.5034	3.1034			
$n = 2000$											
1	True	(2)	(2)	(1.5)	(0)	(1.5)	(−5)	(10)	(0.6)	0.4	0.2
	Mean	2.0016	2.0131	1.4115	0.0155	1.3480	-4.8421	9.5234	0.6010	0.4332	0.1901
	SD	0.0735	0.0415	0.1268	0.0586	0.1000	0.7606	1.4796	0.0123	0.0344	0.0115
	IM SD	0.0739	0.0412	0.0565	0.0500	0.0558	0.8059	1.6752	0.0120	0.0378	0.0156
2	True	(−4)	(−3)	(1.5)	(0)	(1.5)	(−5)	(10)			
	Mean	−3.9930	−2.9772	1.3828	0.0223	1.3009	−4.7825	9.3697			
	SD	0.0904	0.0509	0.1301	0.0750	0.1382	0.9776	1.8163			
	IM SD	0.0943	0.0528	0.0509	0.0674	0.0692	0.9306	1.9150			

Table 5.3 The estimated standard errors for EM parameters of the FM-SN and FM-ST distributions with the *gradient* (*Grad.*), *Hessian* (*Hess.*), and *standard deviation of the sample estimates* (*SD.*) of 1000 samples of size 500, 1000, 2000, and 5000, respectively

		Parameter						
Dist.	Method	μ_1	μ_2	σ_{11}	σ_{22}	λ_1	λ_2	p
$n = 500$								
FM-SN	Grad.	0.4684	0.6224	1.2000	2.1514	1.0337	0.4419	0.0179
	Hess.	0.5000	0.5702	1.2842	2.0084	1.0357	0.4768	0.0179
	SD	0.4125	1.3914	0.9212	1.0888	0.8850	0.8282	0.0175
FM-ST	Grad.	0.3826	0.7392	1.8571	1.5757	1.2713	0.4328	0.0193
	Hess.	0.3937	0.6757	1.9153	1.7518	1.2960	0.4280	0.0197
	SD	0.4190	0.9890	2.5511	2.0463	1.4508	0.5746	0.0192
$n = 1000$								
FM-SN	Grad.	0.2997	0.4348	0.8088	1.4946	0.6465	0.3285	0.0127
	Hess.	0.3425	0.4063	0.9010	1.4203	0.6950	0.3101	0.0126
	SD	0.2543	1.1872	0.7167	0.7943	0.5668	0.6909	0.0125
FM-ST	Grad.	0.2595	0.5178	1.2541	1.0446	0.7926	0.2942	0.0136
	Hess.	0.2655	0.5161	1.2413	1.1336	0.8139	0.3051	0.0137
	SD	0.3078	0.7109	1.7824	1.5037	0.9615	0.4145	0.0138
$n = 2000$								
FM-SN	Grad.	0.2080	0.3006	0.5566	1.0412	0.4296	0.2267	0.0089
	Hess.	0.2365	0.2885	0.6230	1.0141	0.4683	0.2194	0.0089
	SD	0.1873	0.9303	0.5424	0.6130	0.4042	0.5357	0.0089
FM-ST	Grad.	0.1778	0.3509	0.8972	0.7508	0.5543	0.1997	0.0097
	Hess.	0.1891	0.4428	0.9470	0.9934	0.5710	0.2574	0.0100
	SD	0.2289	0.4792	1.3408	1.0227	0.7237	0.2787	0.0104
$n = 5000$								
FM-SN	Grad.	0.1274	0.1808	0.3444	0.6411	0.2601	0.1382	0.0057
	Hess.	0.1439	0.1817	0.3855	0.6482	0.2854	0.1393	0.0057
	SD	0.1340	0.3204	0.3811	0.3483	0.2750	0.1864	0.0053
FM-ST	Grad.	0.1089	0.2170	0.5628	0.4812	0.3404	0.1236	0.0061
	Hess.	0.1139	0.2954	0.6121	0.6384	0.3510	0.1682	0.0063
	SD	0.1639	0.2745	0.9043	0.5783	0.4831	0.1624	0.0066

As we can see in Table 5.3, the results returned by all methods are very similar and improve as n increases. Such results reinforce our belief that the gradient method provides a very good approximation to the asymptotic covariance matrix. Moreover, the gradient method is computationally feasible and easily expandable to the multi-dimensional setup.

Number of Mixture Components

Someone can argue that an arbitrary multivariate density can always be approximated by a finite mixture of normal multivariate distributions, see McLachlan and Peel (2000, Chapter 1), for example. Thus, an interesting comparison can be made if we consider a sample from a two-component mixture of SMSN densities and use some model choice criteria to compare this model with normal mixture models with several number of components.

Here we consider 100 samples of size 2000 from an FM-ST model with two components and parameter values given by (5.8). For model selection, we considered the Akaike information criterion (AIC), the Bayesian information criterion (BIC) and the efficient determination criterion (EDC), defined in Chap. 3.

We fit, besides the true model, the FM-NOR model with 2, 3, and 4 components. Not surprisingly, for all samples, all criteria (see Fig. 5.2) favor the true model, that is, the FM-ST with two components. It is important to emphasize that the FM-NOR models with 3 and 4 components have 17 and 23 parameters, respectively, while the FM-ST model with two components has 16 parameters. Figure 5.2 shows the BIC criterion values for each sample and model. FM-NOR(j) denotes a model with j components.

5.4.3 *Model Fit and Clustering*

Now we illustrate the ability of the FM-SMSN models in fitting data with a known mixture structure not in the FM-SMSN family. Two data sets (FMNT and FMNIG) with different distribution patterns are generated. The FMNT data set is a random sample of size 1000 artificially generated from a mixture of an $\mathrm{N}_2((2,2)^\top, 4\mathbf{I}_2)$ distribution (blue points in Fig. 5.3a) with a $\mathrm{t}_2(\mathbf{0}, 2\mathbf{I}_2, 2)$ distribution.

Several SMSN models were fitted and the resulting model selection criteria values are shown in Table 5.4. EDC1 is the same EDC criterion of the previous section. EDC2 is another version, with $c_n = \log\log n$ in Eq. (4.11). For each model, the algorithm was run 100 times. For each run, the initial value for the location parameter μ_{ji} was generated from a uniform distribution on the interval defined by the range of the observed data in the ith dimension and the initial values for the dispersion matrixes and skewness vectors are fixed as $\mathbf{I}_2$ and $\mathbf{0}$, respectively. A similar strategy was used before by Karlis and Santourian (2009). The results correspond to the solution with the highest log-likelihood. Due to the high computational cost, we considered in the FM-SSL case that ν is a known parameter, fixed at the value 2.

We can see that, despite the symmetrical nature of the mixture components, the normal mixture model poorly fits the data. The skew-normal mixture also has a disappointing performance, because of the heavy-tailed behavior of the data. The SMSN models FM-T and FM-CN show relatively satisfactory results, but is interesting to note that the criteria do not favor them when comparing with their

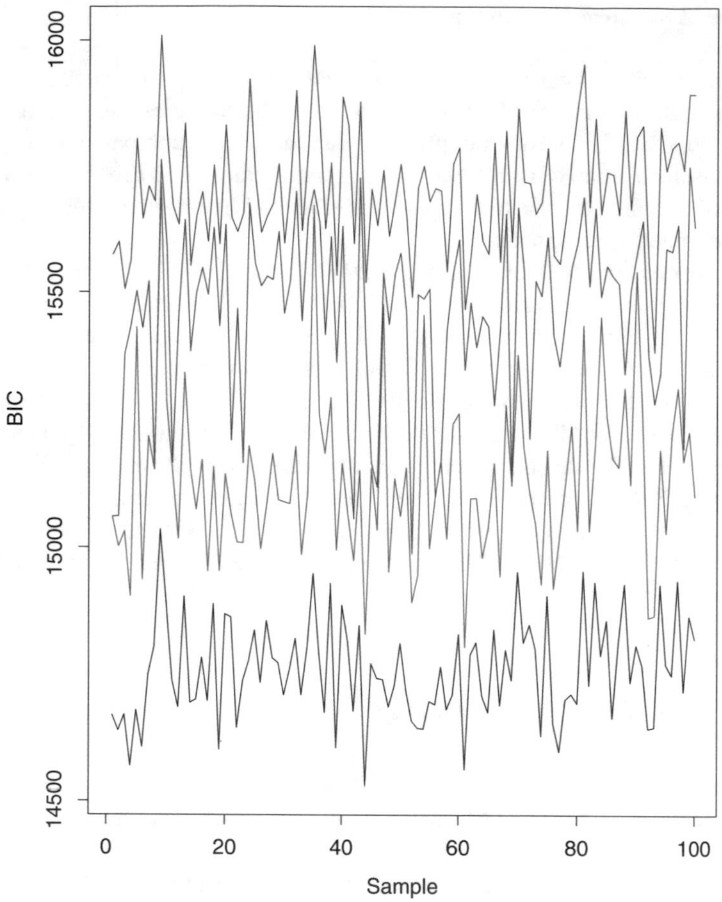

Fig. 5.2 BIC criterion values for 100 samples. Red line: FM-NOR(2), blue line: FM-NOR(3), pink line: FM-NOR(4), black line: FM-ST(2)

asymmetrical counterparts, as one might expect. Also, two of the criteria favored the FM-SCN model when comparing with the FM-T model, with close results when comparing with the FM-ST model. This fact reveals some evidence of the flexibility of the FM-SMSN family. To confirm the usefulness of the skew heavy-tailed models, suppose that the likelihood ratio test is subject to the usual chi-square approximation. Then, we can perform a test of the hypothesis $\boldsymbol{\lambda}_1 = \boldsymbol{\lambda}_2 = \mathbf{0}$ for the FM-ST model, for example. In this case the p-value is 4.563e−06, strongly rejecting it.

In the second experiment, the FMNIG data set is a random sample of size 500 artificially generated from a mixture of two normal inverse Gaussian (NIG) distributions (Karlis and Santourian 2009), see Fig. 5.3b. The parameter values were chosen in order to present a considerable proportion of outliers and skewness pattern

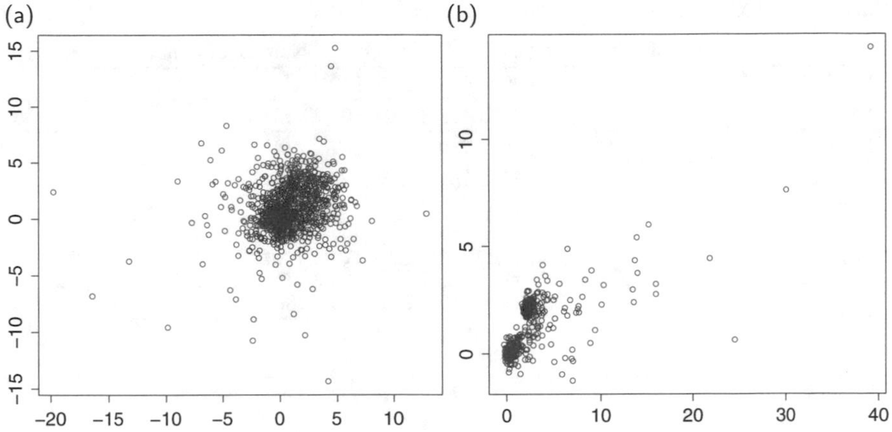

Fig. 5.3 Artificial samples: (**a**) normal and Student-t components and (**b**) NIG components

Table 5.4 Model selection criteria for the FMNT data set

Model	Number of parameters	Log-likelihood	Criterion BIC	EDC1	EDC2	AIC
FM-NOR	11	4345.043	8766.071	8759.656	8711.345	8712.086
FM-T	12	−4288.741	8660.376	8653.377	8600.740	8601.483
FM-SL	12	−4296.258	8675.410	8668.411	8615.708	8618.517
FM-CN	13	−4288.696	8667.192	8659.610	8602.516	8603.391
FM-SN	15	−4328.676	8760.968	8752.220	8686.342	8687.382
FM-ST	16	−4273.667	**8657.857**	**8648.526**	**8578.255**	**8579.333**
FM-SSL ($\nu = 2$)	16	−4277.553	8665.530	8656.300	8586.029	8587.106
FM-SCN	17	**−4273.114**	8663.660	8653.745	8579.083	8580.228

The bold values indicates the best fitting model

and to guarantee a homogeneous covariance structure for the components. The initial values strategy is the *random starts* method suggested by McLachlan and Peel (2000, Sec. 2.12.2).

Here we proceed an unsupervised classification of the points in two groups, ignoring the known true classification, by computing $\hat{z}_{ij}$, the estimated posterior probability that observation i, $(i = 1, \ldots, 500)$ belongs to group j, $(j = 1, 2)$, which is (5.5) evaluated at the EM estimates. If $\hat{z}_{ij} > 1/2$, then $\mathbf{y}_i$ is classified into group j. Obviously, one expects the best classification rate when modeling with NIG components, but it is interesting to verify what happens when we use SMSN components.

Table 5.5 shows the number of right allocations—the clustering performance is measured by choosing among the two possible permutations of group labels the one that yields the highest value. Also are reported the values for the ICL model choice

Table 5.5 Right allocations for the FMNIG data set

Model	Number of parameters	BIC	ICL	Number of right allocations
FM-NOR	11	2991.676	3020.310	292
FM-T	12	2483.423	2556.100	456
FM-CN	13	2671.739	2753.167	478
FM-SL ($\nu = 0.7$)	12	2538.134	2589.898	456
FM-SN	15	2776.672	2822.427	276
FM-ST	16	2223.219	2291.225	**485**
FM-SCN	17	2369.219	2425.413	480
FM-SSL ($\nu = 0.7$)	16	2257.574	2316.791	482
FM-SN ($\mathbf{\Gamma}_1 = \mathbf{\Gamma}_2$)	12	2911.776	2976.092	276
FM-ST ($\mathbf{\Gamma}_1 = \mathbf{\Gamma}_2$)	13	**2207.395**	**2275.011**	483
FM-SCN ($\mathbf{\Gamma}_1 = \mathbf{\Gamma}_2$)	14	2357.845	2429.544	481

The bold values indicates the best fitting model

criterion (Biernacki et al. 2000; Basso et al. 2010). This is suitable for classification purposes because it penalizes model complexity (like AIC, BIC, and EDC) and the inability of the fitted mixture model to provide a reasonable partition of the data. This inability is measured by the difference between ICL and BIC, which is the *estimated mean entropy*. A curious fact, captured by this measure, is that when comparing FM-SN with FM-NOR, the ICL favors the former but the number of right allocations is greater for the latter.

Note also from Table 5.5 that the FM-ST model with equal dispersion matrixes ($\mathbf{\Gamma}_1 = \mathbf{\Gamma}_2$) presents the best fit, which is not surprising because of the homogeneous nature of the covariance structure.

We also have conducted similar experiments with dimensions and number of components greater than two, but the results were similar to that already presented. The choice of two dimensions has the advantage of giving us an appealing graphical representation of the components, as depicted in Fig. 5.3.

5.4.4 The Pima Indians Diabetes Data

The *Pima Indians Diabetes* is a benchmark data set for binary classifications. The main goal is to decide whether a subject has diabetes or not, based on eight measured variables. Data can be freely downloaded from the UCI Machine Learning Repository (Frank and Asuncion 2010). We removed subjects with missing values and the variables triceps and insulin, which are missing for most subjects, resulting in a reduced set with 724 individuals. The usual analysis of this data set is from the *supervised classification* point of view, where classification of new subjects is made based on learning from a training data set. Similar to the analysis of the previous section, here we consider, besides the model fit issue, only the (unsupervised) clustering of the observations in two groups. All the subjects in this set have a correct diagnostic, allowing us to count the number of right classifications.

The results of the estimation procedure for some FM-SMSN models (using the random starts strategy) are presented in Table 5.6. All the criteria favors the models with specific skewed/heavy-tailed components (FM-ST, FM-SSL, and FM-SCN) when comparing with models with symmetric components (FM-NOR and FM-T) or even with the FM-SN model. From the clustering point of view, in order to give stronger evidence of the superiority of the method using the FM-SMSN family, we proceeded a bootstrap experiment with 1500 replications. For each replication, the right number of allocations was computed. The mean and sample deviance values of these bootstrap replications are shown in Table 5.7. Also, we present the associated 95% normal asymptotic confidence intervals. We can see that the means are greater and the standard deviations are smaller for the skewed/heavy-tailed FM-SMSN models (except for the case with equal dispersion matrixes), confirming our expectations.

We emphasize that the clustering approach based on the FM-SMSN family presented here can be seen as a starting point of a more detailed one, since more

Table 5.6 Model selection criteria for the Pima Indians Diabetes data set

		Criterion				
Model	log-likelihood	BIC	EDC1	EDC2	AIC	ICL
FM-NOR	−13023.540	26409.240	26150.740	26343.060	26157.080	26483.970
FM-T	−13009.800	26388.340	26125.140	26320.950	26131.590	26452.290
FM-SN	−12838.900	26118.990	25804.090	26038.360	25811.810	26212.540
FM-ST	−12824.840	26097.440	25777.840	26015.610	25785.680	26180.770
FM-SSL	−12823.670	26095.110	25775.500	26013.280	25783.340	26197.670
FM-SCN	**−12820.080**	**26094.500**	**25770.200**	**26011.470**	**25778.150**	**26202.660**
FM-ST ($\boldsymbol{\Gamma}_1 = \boldsymbol{\Gamma}_2$)	−13074.200	26457.880	26236.980	26401.320	26242.390	26494.470

The bold values indicates the best fitting model

Table 5.7 Right allocations analysis through bootstrap procedure for the Pima Indians Diabetes data set

Model	Mean of right allocations	Standard deviation of right allocations	95% confidence interval for right allocations
FM-NOR	512.288	25.225	(462.846, 561.730)
FM-T	508.924	23.470	(462.922, 554.926)
FM-SN	520.461	18.529	(484.144, 556.777)
FM-ST	519.535	18.159	(483.944, 555.126)
FM-SSL	533.559	17.973	(498.333, 568.785)
FM-SCN	520.402	18.762	(483.628, 557.176)
FM-ST ($\boldsymbol{\Gamma}_1 = \boldsymbol{\Gamma}_2$)	530.861	31.172	(469.763,591.958)

elaborated methodologies can be developed using this framework. For example, it would be interesting to explore a skew extension of the *mixture of factor analyzers model* suggested by McLachlan et al. (2007).

5.5 Identifiability and Unboundedness

Modeling based on finite mixture models is a research area with several challenging aspects. There are nontrivial issues, not considered in this work, which deserve a more detailed investigation.

First, we comment about identifiability. The class of FM-SMSN models will be identifiable if distinct component densities correspond to distinct mixtures. More specifically, if we have two representations for the same mixture distribution, say

$$\sum_{j=1}^{G} p'_j g(\cdot|\boldsymbol{\mu}'_j, \boldsymbol{\Sigma}'_j, \boldsymbol{\lambda}'_j, \boldsymbol{\nu}) = \sum_{j=1}^{G} p_j g(\cdot|\boldsymbol{\mu}_j, \boldsymbol{\Sigma}_j, \boldsymbol{\lambda}_j, \boldsymbol{\nu}),$$

then

$$p'_j = p_{\rho(j)}, \quad \boldsymbol{\mu}'_j = \boldsymbol{\mu}_{\rho(j)}, \quad \boldsymbol{\Sigma}'_j = \boldsymbol{\Sigma}_{\rho(j)}, \quad \boldsymbol{\lambda}'_j = \boldsymbol{\lambda}_{\rho(j)}$$

for some permutation ρ of the indexes $1, \ldots, G$ (Titterington et al. 1985, Chapter 3). Considering specific members of the FM-SMSN family, the FM-NOR identifiability was first verified by Yakowitz and Spragins (1968), but previous discussions in the related literature concerning the FM-T model—see references in Sect. 5.1—do not present a formal proof of its identifiability.

Holzmann et al. (2006) have established the identifiability of finite mixtures of elliptical distributions under conditions on the characteristic or density generators. FM-NOR and FM-T models belong to this family. They also show conditions on the mixing distribution H in order to guarantee identifiability of some members of finite mixtures of SMN distributions. Obviously, it is of interest to extend these results to the FM-SMSN family, mainly because the recent literature involving mixtures of skew distributions—see Sect. 5.1 again—do not present formal discussions about this theme.

The mixture likelihood is unbounded—see commentaries in Sect. 5.2.1—and may present local spurious maxima and singularities. Thus, another topic of interest is the constrained optimization of the likelihood. This was done for the univariate FM-NOR model by Hathaway (1985), where conditions on the component variances were imposed in order to obtain global maximization. The consistency of the resulting estimator is also proved. This work had a considerable expansion in the sequence of papers Ingrassia (2004), Ingrassia and Rocci (2007) and Greselin and Ingrassia (2010), the first two dealing with the multivariate FM-NOR model and the last with the multivariate FM-T model.

Chapter 6
Mixture Regression Modeling Based on SMSN Distributions

The traditional estimation of mixture regression models is based on the assumption of normality (symmetry) of component errors and thus is sensitive to outliers, heavy-tailed errors and/or asymmetric errors. In this chapter we present a proposal to deal with these issues simultaneously in the context of the mixture regression by extending the classic normal model by assuming that the random errors follow a scale mixtures of skew-normal distributions. This approach allows us to model data with great flexibility, accommodating skewness and heavy tails. The main virtue of considering the mixture regression models under the class of scale mixtures of skew-normal distributions is that they have a nice hierarchical representation which allows easy implementation of inference. We develop a simple EM-type algorithm to perform maximum likelihood inference of the parameters of the proposed model. The presentation is mainly based on Zeller et al. (2016), extending the works of Yao et al. (2014), which is a mixture regression using the Student-t distribution, and Liu and Lin (2014) who proposed a mixture regression by using the skew-normal model.

6.1 Introduction

In applied statistics, a large number of applications deal with relating a random variable Y_i, which is observed on several occasions $i = 1, \ldots, n$, to a set of explanatory variables or covariates $(x_{i1}, \ldots, x_{id-1})$ through a regression-type model, where the conditional mean of Y_i is assumed to depend on $\mathbf{x}_i = (1 \ x_{i1} \ldots x_{id-1})^\top$ through $\mathrm{E}[Y_i|\boldsymbol{\beta}, \mathbf{x}_i] = \mathbf{x}_i^\top \boldsymbol{\beta}$, where $\boldsymbol{\beta}$ is a vector of unknown regression coefficients of dimension d. In many circumstances, however, the assumption that the regression coefficient is fixed over all possible realizations of $Y_1, \ldots, Y_n$ is inadequate, and models where the regression coefficient changes are of great practical importance. One way to capture such changes in the parameter of a regression model is

V. H. Lachos Dávila et al., *Finite Mixture of Skewed Distributions*,
SpringerBriefs in Statistics, https://doi.org/10.1007/978-3-319-98029-4_6

to use finite mixtures of regression models (MRM). MRM are widely used to investigate the relationship between variables coming from several unknown latent homogeneous groups. They were first introduced by Quandt (1972) under the titles *switching regression* or *clusterwise linear regression* (Späth 1979). Comprehensive surveys are available in McLachlan and Peel (2000), and from a Bayesian point of view, in Frühwirth-Schnatter (2006, chap. 8).

The literature on maximum likelihood estimation of the parameters of the Gaussian MRM (hereafter N-MRM) is very extensive. Applications include marketing (DeSarbo and Cron 1988; DeSarbo et al. 1992; Quandt and Ramsey 1978), economics (Cosslett and Lee 1985; Hamilton 1989), agriculture (Turner 2000), nutrition (Arellano-Valle et al. 2008), and psychometrics (Liu et al. 2011). The standard algorithm in this case is the so-called EM (Expectation-Maximization) of Dempster et al. (1977), or perhaps some extension like the ECM (Meng and Rubin 1993) or the ECME (Liu and Rubin 1994) algorithms. Many extensions of this classic model have been proposed to broaden the applicability of linear regression analysis to situations where the Gaussian error term assumption may be inadequate, for example, because the datasets involve skewed or longer than normal tails errors. Some such extensions rely on the use of the skew-normal (Azzalini 1985) and the Student-t distributions, respectively. An MRM based on the Student-t model (T-MRM) has been recently proposed by Yao et al. (2014) to estimate the mixture regression parameters robustly. Liu and Lin (2014) proposed a robust version of the MRM by using the skew-normal model (SN-MRM), which appears to be a more theoretically compelling modeling tool for practitioners because it can investigate differential effects of covariates and accommodate moderately asymmetrical errors.

In this chapter, we propose a unified robust mixture regression model based on scale mixtures of skew-normal distributions by extending the mixture of scale mixtures of skew-normal distributions proposed by Basso et al. (2010) to the regression setting. As observed before, the class of SMSN distributions, proposed by Branco and Dey (2001), is attractive since it simultaneously models skewness and heavy tails. Besides this, it has a stochastic representation for easy implementation of the EM algorithm and it also facilitates the study of many useful properties. This extension results in a flexible class of models for robust estimation in MRM since it contains distributions such as the skew-normal distribution and all the symmetric class of scale mixtures of normal distributions defined by Andrews and Mallows (1974). Moreover, the class of SMSN distributions is a rich class that contains proper elements such as the skew-t (Azzalini and Capitanio 2003), skew-slash (Wang and Genton 2006), and skew-contaminated normal distribution (Lachos et al. 2010). Therefore they can be used in many types of models to infer robustness. In addition, this rich class of distributions can naturally attribute different weights to each observation and consequently control the influence of a single observation on the parameter estimates. Thus, the objectives of this chapter are: (1) to propose a mixture regression estimation method based on SMSN distributions, extending the recent works of Yao et al. (2014) and Liu and Lin (2014) (see also Doğru and Arslan 2017); (2) to implement and evaluate the proposed method computationally; and (3) to apply these results to the analysis of a real life dataset.

The remainder of the chapter is organized as follows. In Sect. 6.2, we present the SMSN-MRM, including the EM algorithm for maximum likelihood (ML) estimation. In Sects. 6.3 and 6.4, numerical examples using both simulated and real data are given to illustrate the performance of the proposed method.

6.2 The Proposed Model

In this section, we consider the mixture regression model where the random errors follow a scale mixtures of skew-normal distributions (SMSN-MRM). In general, a normal mixture regression model (N-MRM) is defined as: let Z be a latent class variable such that given $Z = j$, the response Y depends on the p-dimensional predictor $\mathbf{x}$ in a linear way

$$Y = \mathbf{x}^\top \boldsymbol{\beta}_j + \epsilon_j, \quad j = 1, \ldots, G, \tag{6.1}$$

where G is the number of groups (also called components in mixture models) in the population and $\epsilon_j \sim N(0, \sigma_j^2)$ is independent of $\mathbf{x}$. Suppose that $P(Z = j) = p_j$ and Z is independent of $\mathbf{x}$, then the conditional density of Y given $\mathbf{x}$, without observing Z, is

$$f(y|\mathbf{x}, \boldsymbol{\theta}) = \sum_{j=1}^{G} p_j \phi(y|\mathbf{x}^\top \boldsymbol{\beta}_j, \sigma_j^2), \tag{6.2}$$

where $\boldsymbol{\theta} = (\boldsymbol{\theta}_1^\top, \ldots, \boldsymbol{\theta}_G^\top)^\top$, with $\boldsymbol{\theta}_j = (p_j, \boldsymbol{\beta}_j^\top, \sigma_j^2)^\top$. The model (6.2) is the so-called normal mixture of regression models. Following Yao et al. (2014) and Liu and Lin (2014), we extend the N-MRM defined above by considering the linear relationship in (6.1) with the following assumption:

$$\epsilon_j \sim \text{SMSN}(b\Delta_j, \sigma_j^2, \lambda_j, \boldsymbol{\nu}_j), \quad j = 1, \ldots, G, \tag{6.3}$$

where $\Delta_j = \sigma_j \delta_j$, $\delta_j = \dfrac{\lambda_j}{\sqrt{1 + \lambda_j^2}}$, $b = -\sqrt{\frac{2}{\pi}} K_1$, with $K_r = E[U^{-r/2}]$, $r = 1, 2, \ldots$, which corresponds to the regression model where the error distribution has mean zero and hence the regression parameters are all comparable.

The mixture regression model with scale mixtures of skew-normal distributions defined above can be formulated in a similar way to the model defined in (6.2) as follows:

$$f(y|\mathbf{x}, \boldsymbol{\theta}) = \sum_{j=1}^{G} p_j g(y|\mathbf{x}, \boldsymbol{\theta}_j), \tag{6.4}$$

where $g(\cdot|\mathbf{x}, \boldsymbol{\theta}_j)$ is the density function of SMSN$(\mathbf{x}^\top\boldsymbol{\beta}_j + b\Delta_j, \sigma_j^2, \lambda_j, \boldsymbol{\nu}_j)$ and $\boldsymbol{\theta}_j = (p_j, \boldsymbol{\beta}_j^\top, \sigma_j^2, \lambda_j, \boldsymbol{\nu}_j)^\top$. Concerning the parameter $\boldsymbol{\nu}_j$ of the mixing distribution $H(; \boldsymbol{\nu}_j)$, for $j = 1, \ldots, G$, it can be a vector of parameters, e.g., the contaminated normal distribution. For computational convenience we assume that $\boldsymbol{\nu} = \boldsymbol{\nu}_1 = \boldsymbol{\nu}_2 = \ldots, \boldsymbol{\nu}_G$. This strategy works very well in the empirical studies that we have conducted and greatly simplifies the optimization problem. Observe that the model considers that the regression coefficient and the error variance are not homogeneous over all independent possible pairs $(Y_i, \mathbf{x}_i)$, $i = 1 \ldots, n$. In fact, they change between subgroups of observations.

In the context of classic inference, the unknown parameter $\boldsymbol{\theta}$, given observations $(\mathbf{x}_1, y_1), \ldots, (\mathbf{x}_n, y_n)$, is traditionally estimated by the maximum likelihood estimate (MLE):

$$\widehat{\boldsymbol{\theta}} = \arg\max_{\boldsymbol{\theta}} \sum_{i=1}^{n} \log(f(y_i|\mathbf{x}_i, \boldsymbol{\theta})). \tag{6.5}$$

Note that the maximizer of (6.5) does not have an explicit solution, so we propose to use an EM-type algorithm (Dempster et al. 1977). For a gentle tutorial on the EM algorithm and its applications to parameter estimation for mixture models, see McLachlan and Peel (2000).

6.2.1 Maximum Likelihood Estimation via EM Algorithm

In this section, we present an EM algorithm for the ML estimation of the mixture regression model with scale mixtures of skew-normal distributions. To explore the EM algorithm we present the SMSN-MRM in an incomplete-data framework, using the results presented in Chap. 2.

As in (2.1), in order to simplify notations, algebra, and future interpretations, it is appropriate to deal with a random vector $\mathbf{Z}_i = (Z_{i1}, \ldots, Z_{iG})^\top$ instead of the random variable Z_i, where

$$Z_{ij} = \begin{cases} 1, & \text{if the ith observation is from the jth component;} \\ 0, & \text{otherwise.} \end{cases}$$

Consequently, under this approach the random vector $\mathbf{Z}_i \overset{\text{iid}}{\sim} \text{Multinomial}(1; p_1, \ldots, p_g)$, such that

$$Y_i|Z_{ij} = 1 \overset{\text{ind}}{\sim} \text{SMSN}(\mathbf{x}_i^\top\boldsymbol{\beta}_j + b\Delta_j, \sigma_j^2, \lambda_j, \boldsymbol{\nu}_j).$$

Observe that $Z_{ij} = 1$ if and only if $Z_i = j$. Thus, the setup defined above, along with (3.18)–(3.20), can be written hierarchically as

$$Y_i|T_i = t_i, U_i = u_i, Z_{ij} = 1 \overset{\text{ind}}{\sim} \mathrm{N}(\mathbf{x}_i^\top \boldsymbol{\beta}_j + \Delta_j t_i, u_i^{-1}\Gamma_j), \tag{6.6}$$

$$T_i|U_i = u_i, Z_{ij} = 1 \overset{\text{iid}}{\sim} \mathrm{TN}_1(b, u_i^{-1}; (b, \infty)), \tag{6.7}$$

$$U_i|Z_{ij} = 1 \overset{\text{ind}}{\sim} H(u_i; \boldsymbol{\nu}), \tag{6.8}$$

$$\mathbf{Z}_i \overset{\text{iid}}{\sim} \text{Multinomial}(1; p_1, \ldots, p_g), \tag{6.9}$$

for $i = 1, \ldots, n$, all independent, where $\Gamma_j = \sigma_j^2 - \Delta_j^2$ and $\mathrm{TN}_1(r, s; (a, b))$ denotes the univariate normal distribution ($\mathrm{N}(r, s)$), truncated on the interval (a, b). Let $\mathbf{y} = (y_1, \ldots, y_n)^\top$, $\mathbf{u} = (u_1, \ldots, u_n)^\top$, $\mathbf{t} = (t_1, \ldots, t_n)^\top$, and $\mathbf{z} = (\mathbf{z}_1^\top, \ldots, \mathbf{z}_n^\top)^\top$. Then, under the hierarchical representation (6.6)–(6.9), it follows that the complete log-likelihood function associated with $\mathbf{y}_c = (\mathbf{y}^\top, \mathbf{u}^\top, \mathbf{t}^\top, \mathbf{z}^\top)^\top$ is

$$\ell_c(\boldsymbol{\theta}|\mathbf{y}_c) = c + \sum_{i=1}^{n}\sum_{j=1}^{G} z_{ij}\left[\log p_j - \frac{1}{2}\log\Gamma_j\right.$$
$$\left. - \frac{1}{2\Gamma_j} u_i (y_i - \mathbf{x}_i^\top \boldsymbol{\beta}_j - \Delta_j t_i)^2 + \log(h(u_i; \boldsymbol{\nu}))\right],$$

where c is a constant that is independent of the parameter vector $\boldsymbol{\theta}$ and $h(\cdot; \boldsymbol{\nu})$ is the density of U_i.

Let $\widehat{\boldsymbol{\theta}}_j^{(k)} = (\widehat{p}_j^{(k)}, \widehat{\boldsymbol{\beta}}_j^{(k)\top}, \widehat{\sigma^2}_j^{(k)}, \widehat{\lambda}_j^{(k)}, \boldsymbol{\nu}^{(k)})^\top$ be the estimates of $\boldsymbol{\theta}$ at the k-th iteration. It follows, after some simple algebra, that the conditional expectation of the complete log-likelihood function has the form

$$Q(\boldsymbol{\theta}|\widehat{\boldsymbol{\theta}}^{(k)}) = c + \sum_{i=1}^{n}\sum_{j=1}^{G} \widehat{z}_{ij}^{(k)} \log p_j - \frac{1}{2}\sum_{i=1}^{n}\sum_{j=1}^{G} \widehat{z}_{ij}^{(k)} \log\Gamma_j$$
$$- \frac{1}{2}\sum_{i=1}^{n}\sum_{j=1}^{G} \frac{\widehat{zu}_{ij}^{(k)}}{\Gamma_j}(y_i - \mathbf{x}_i^\top \boldsymbol{\beta}_j)^2$$
$$+ \sum_{i=1}^{n}\sum_{j=1}^{G} \frac{\widehat{zut}_{ij}^{(k)}}{\Gamma_j}(y_i - \mathbf{x}_i^\top \boldsymbol{\beta}_j)\Delta_j - \frac{1}{2}\sum_{i=1}^{n}\sum_{j=1}^{G} \frac{\widehat{zut^2}_{ij}^{(k)}}{\Gamma_j}\Delta_j^2,$$

where $\widehat{z}_{ij}^{(k)} = E[Z_{ij}|y_i, \widehat{\boldsymbol{\theta}}^{(k)}]$, $\widehat{zu}_{ij}^{(k)} = E[Z_{ij}U_i|y_i, \widehat{\boldsymbol{\theta}}^{(k)}]$, $\widehat{zut}_{ij}^{(k)} = E[Z_{ij}U_iT_i|y_i, \widehat{\boldsymbol{\theta}}^{(k)}]$, and $\widehat{zut^2}_{ij}^{(k)} = E[Z_{ij}U_iT_i^2|y_i, \widehat{\boldsymbol{\theta}}^{(k)}]$. By using known properties of conditional expectation, we obtain

$$\widehat{z}_{ij}^{(k)} = \frac{\widehat{p}_j^{(k)} g(y_i|\mathbf{x}_i, \widehat{\boldsymbol{\theta}}_j^{(k)})}{\sum_{j=1}^{G} \widehat{p}_j^{(k)} g(y_i|\mathbf{x}_i, \widehat{\boldsymbol{\theta}}_j^{(k)})}, \tag{6.10}$$

$\widehat{zu}_{ij}^{(k)} = \widehat{z}_{ij}^{(k)} \widehat{u}_{ij}^{(k)}$, $\widehat{zut}_{ij}^{(k)} = \widehat{z}_{ij}^{(k)} \widehat{ut}_{ij}^{(k)}$ and $\widehat{zut^2}_{ij}^{(k)} = \widehat{z}_{ij}^{(k)} \widehat{ut^2}_{ij}^{(k)}$, with

$$\widehat{ut}_{ij}^{(k)} = \widehat{u}_{ij}^{(k)} (\widehat{m}_{ij}^{(k)} + b) + \widehat{M}_j^{(k)} \widehat{\eta}_{ij}^{(k)}, \tag{6.11}$$

$$\widehat{ut^2}_{ij}^{(k)} = \widehat{u}_{ij}^{(k)} (\widehat{m}_{ij}^{(k)} + b)^2 + \widehat{M}_j^{2(k)} + \widehat{M}_j^{(k)} (\widehat{m}_{ij}^{(k)} + 2b) \widehat{\eta}_{ij}^{(k)}, \tag{6.12}$$

where $\widehat{M}_j^2 = \dfrac{\widehat{\Gamma}_j}{\widehat{\Gamma}_j + \widehat{\Delta}_j^2}$ and $\widehat{m}_{ij} = \widehat{M}_j^2 \dfrac{\widehat{\Delta}_j}{\widehat{\Gamma}_j}(y_i - \mathbf{x}_i^\top \widehat{\boldsymbol{\beta}}_j - b\widehat{\Delta}_j)$, $i = 1, \ldots, n$, with all these quantities evaluated at $\boldsymbol{\theta} = \widehat{\boldsymbol{\theta}}^{(k)}$. Since $a_{ij} = \dfrac{m_{ij}}{M_{ij}} = \lambda_j \sigma_j (y_i - \mathbf{x}_i^\top \boldsymbol{\beta}_j - b\Delta_j)$, the conditional expectations given in (6.11)–(6.12), specifically $\widehat{u}_{ij}$ and $\widehat{\eta}_{ij}$, can be easily derived from the result given in Sect. 3.3.1. Thus, at least for the ST and SCN distributions, we have a closed-form expression for the quantities $\widehat{u}_{ij}$ and $\widehat{\eta}_{ij}$, as can be found in Zeller et al. (2011) and Basso et al. (2010). For the SSL, Monte Carlo integration can be employed, which yields the so-called MC-EM algorithm; see Wei and Tanner (1990), McLachlan and Krishnan (2008), and Zeller et al. (2011).

Also, we have adopted the same strategy used in Chaps. 3 and 4 to update the estimate of $\boldsymbol{\nu}$, by direct maximization of the marginal log-likelihood.

Thus, the ECME algorithm for maximum likelihood estimation of $\boldsymbol{\theta}$ is defined as follows:

E-step: Given $\boldsymbol{\theta} = \widehat{\boldsymbol{\theta}}^{(k)}$, compute $\widehat{z}_{ij}^{(k)}$, $\widehat{zu}_{ij}^{(k)}$, $\widehat{zut}_{ij}^{(k)}$, and $\widehat{zut^2}_{ij}^{(k)}$, for $i = 1, \ldots, n$, using (6.11)–(6.12).

CM-step: Update $\widehat{\boldsymbol{\theta}}^{(k+1)}$ by maximizing $Q(\boldsymbol{\theta}|\widehat{\boldsymbol{\theta}}^{(k)})$ over $\boldsymbol{\theta}$, which leads to the following closed form expressions:

$$\widehat{p}_j^{(k+1)} = \frac{\sum_{i=1}^n \widehat{z}_{ij}^{(k)}}{n},$$

$$\widehat{\boldsymbol{\beta}}_j^{(k+1)} = (\sum_{i=1}^n \widehat{zu}_{ij}^{(k)} \mathbf{x}_i \mathbf{x}_i^\top)^{-1} \sum_{i=1}^n (\widehat{zu}_i^{(k)} y_i - \widehat{zut}_{ij}^{(k)} \widehat{\Delta}_j^{(k)}) \mathbf{x}_i,$$

$$\widehat{\Gamma}_j^{(k+1)} = \frac{\sum_{i=1}^n \left[\widehat{zu}_{ij}^{(k)} (y_i - \mathbf{x}_i^\top \widehat{\boldsymbol{\beta}}_j^{(k+1)})^2 - 2\widehat{zut}_{ij}^{(k)} \widehat{\Delta}_j^{(k)} (y_i - \mathbf{x}_i^\top \widehat{\boldsymbol{\beta}}_j^{(k+1)}) + \widehat{zut^2}_{ij}^{(k)} \widehat{\Delta}_j^{2(k)} \right]}{\sum_{i=1}^n \widehat{z}_{ij}^{(k)}},$$

$$\widehat{\Delta}_j^{(k+1)} = \frac{\sum_{i=1}^n \widehat{zut}_{ij}^{(k)} (y_i - \mathbf{x}_i^\top \widehat{\boldsymbol{\beta}}_j^{(k+1)})}{\sum_{i=1}^n \widehat{zut^2}_{ij}^{(k)}},$$

$$\widehat{\sigma^2}_j^{(k+1)} = \widehat{\Gamma}_j^{(k+1)} + \widehat{\Delta}_j^{2(k+1)}, \quad \widehat{\lambda}_j^{(k+1)} = \frac{\widehat{\Delta}_j^{(k+1)}}{\sqrt{\widehat{\Gamma}_j^{(k+1)}}}, \quad j = 1, \ldots, G.$$

CML-step: Update $\widehat{\boldsymbol{\nu}}^{(k)}$ by maximizing the actual marginal log-likelihood function, obtaining

$$\widehat{\boldsymbol{\nu}}^{(k+1)} = \arg\max_{\boldsymbol{\nu}} \sum_{i=1}^{n} \log\left(\sum_{j=1}^{G} \widehat{p}_j^{(k)} g(y_i|\mathbf{x}_i, \widehat{\boldsymbol{\beta}}_j^{(k+1)}, \widehat{\sigma^2}_j^{(k+1)}, \widehat{\boldsymbol{\lambda}}_j^{(k+1)}, \boldsymbol{\nu})\right),$$

where $g(.|\mathbf{x}_i, \boldsymbol{\theta}_j)$ is defined in (6.4).

A more parsimonious model is achieved by supposing $\Gamma_1 = \ldots = \Gamma_G = \Gamma$, which can be seen as an extension of the N-MRM with restricted variance–covariance components. In this case, the updates for $\widehat{p}_j^{(k)}$, $\widehat{\boldsymbol{\beta}}_j^{(k)}$ and $\widehat{\Delta}_j^{(k)}$ remain the same, and the update for $\widehat{\Gamma}_j^{(k)}$ is given by

$$\widehat{\Gamma}^{(k+1)} = \frac{1}{n} \sum_{i=1}^{n} \sum_{j=1}^{G} \widehat{z}_{ij}^{(k)} \widehat{\Gamma}_j^{(k+1)}.$$

The iterations are repeated until a suitable convergence rule is satisfied, e.g.,

$$\left| \frac{\ell(\widehat{\boldsymbol{\theta}}^{(k+1)})}{\ell(\widehat{\boldsymbol{\theta}}^{(k)})} - 1 \right| < 10^{-5}. \tag{6.13}$$

Useful starting values required to implement this algorithm are those obtained under the normality assumption when $\widehat{\lambda}_j^{(0)} = 3\text{sign}(\widehat{\rho}_j)$, where $\widehat{\rho}_j$ is the sample skewness coefficient for group j, for $j = 1, \ldots, G$. However, in order to ensure that the true maximum likelihood estimates are identified, we recommend running the EM algorithm using a range of different starting values. Note that when $\lambda_j = 0$ (or $\Delta_j = 0$) the M-step equations reduce to the equations obtained assuming SMN distributions. Particularly, this algorithm clearly generalizes the results found in Yao et al. (2014) by taking $U_i \sim Gamma(\frac{\nu}{2}, \frac{\nu}{2}), i = 1, \ldots, n$.

6.2.2 Notes on Implementation

It is well known that mixture models may provide a multimodal log-likelihood function. In this sense, the method of maximum likelihood estimation through EM algorithm may not give maximum global solutions if the starting values are far from the real parameter values. Thus, the choice of starting values for the EM algorithm in the mixture context plays a big role in parameter estimation. In our examples and simulation studies we consider the following procedure for the SMSN-MRM.

- Partition the sample into G groups using the K-means clustering algorithm (Basso et al. 2010);

- Compute the proportion of data points belonging to the same cluster j, say $p_j^{(0)}$, $j = 1, \ldots, G$. This is the initial value for p_j;
- For each group j, compute the initial values $\boldsymbol{\beta}_j^{(0)}$ using the method of least squares. Then, use the residuals of each group to compute initial values $(\sigma_j^2)^{(0)}$, $\lambda_j^{(0)}$ and $\nu^{(0)}$ by using the R package *smsnmix()* (Prates et al. 2013).

Because there is no universal criterion for mixture model selection, we chose four criteria to compare the models in the SMSN family. The first three are the Akaike information criterion (AIC), the Bayesian information criterion (BIC), and the efficient determination criterion (EDC), defined in Sect. 4.4.3. We also considered the values of ICL (Integrated Completed Likelihood) choice criterion (Basso et al. 2010) for the models. This is suitable for classification purposes because it penalizes model complexity (like AIC, BIC, and EDC) and the inability of the fitted mixture model to provide a reasonable partition of the data. This inability is measured by the difference between ICL and BIC, which is the estimated mean entropy.

In the next sections, simulation studies and a real dataset are presented in order to illustrate the performance of the proposed method.

6.3 Simulation Experiments

In this section, we consider three simulation experiments to show the applicability of our proposed model. Our intention is to show that the SMSN-MRM can do exactly what it is designed for, that is, satisfactorily model data that have a structure with serious departures from the normal assumption.

6.3.1 Experiment 1: Parameter Recovery

In this section, we consider two scenarios for simulation in order to verify if we can estimate the true parameter values accurately by using the proposed estimation method. This is the first step to ensure that the estimation procedure works satisfactorily. We fit the SMSN-MRM to data that were artificially generated from the following SMSN-MRM:

$$\begin{cases} Y_i = \mathbf{x}_i^\top \boldsymbol{\beta}_1 + \epsilon_1, \ Z_{i1} = 1, \\ Y_i = \mathbf{x}_i^\top \boldsymbol{\beta}_2 + \epsilon_2, \ Z_{i2} = 1, \end{cases}$$

where Z_{ij} is a component indicator of Y_i with $P(Z_{ij} = 1) = p_j, j = 1, 2, \mathbf{x}_i^\top = (1, x_{i1}, x_{i2})$, such that $x_{i1} \sim U(0, 1)$ and $x_{i2} \sim U(-1, 1)$, $i = 1, \ldots, n$, and ϵ_1 and ϵ_2 follow a distribution in the family of SMSN distributions, as the assumption given in (6.3).

We generated 500 random samples of size $n = 500$ from the SN, ST, and the SSL models with the following parameter values: $\boldsymbol{\beta}_1 = (\beta_{01}, \beta_{11}, \beta_{21})^\top =$

$(-1, -4, -3)^\top$, $\boldsymbol{\beta}_2 = (\beta_{02}, \beta_{12}, \beta_{22})^\top = (3, 7, 2)^\top$, $p_1 = 0.3$ and $\nu = 3$. In addition, we consider the following scenarios: scenario 1 : $\sigma_1^2 = 2, \sigma_2^2 = 1, \lambda_1 = 2$ and $\lambda_2 = 4$, and scenario 2 : $\sigma_1^2 = \sigma_2^2 = 2$ and $\lambda_1 = \lambda_2 = 2$, i.e., $\Gamma_1 = \Gamma_2$. We used the maximum likelihood estimation via EM algorithm for each sample, using the stopping criterion (6.13). No existing program is available to estimate SMSN-MRM directly. Therefore, ML estimation via the EM algorithm was implemented using R.

In the mixture context, the likelihood is invariant under a permutation of the class labels in parameter vectors. Therefore, a label switching problem can occur when some labels of the mixture classes permute (McLachlan and Peel 2000). Although the switching of class labels is not a concern in the general course of the maximum likelihood estimation via the EM algorithm for studies with only one replication, it was a serious problem in our simulation study because the same model was estimated iteratively for 500 replications per cell. To solve this problem, we chose the labels by minimizing the distance to the true parameter values. The average values and the corresponding standard deviations (SD) of the EM estimates across all samples were computed and the results are presented in Tables 6.1 and 6.2. Note that all the point estimates are quite accurate in all the considered scenarios. Thus, the results suggest that the proposed EM-type algorithm produced satisfactory estimates.

6.3.2 *Experiment 2: Classification*

In this section, we illustrate the ability of the SMSN-MRM to fit data with a mixture structure generated from a different family of skew distribution and we also

Table 6.1 Scenario 1: mean and standard deviations (SD) for EM estimates based on 500 samples from the SMSN-MRM

	SN		ST		SSL	
Parameter	Mean	SD	Mean	SD	Mean	SD
$\beta_{01}(-1)$	−1.0008	0.1593	−1.0054	0.2358	−0.9902	0.1961
$\beta_{11}(-4)$	−4.0075	0.2640	−3.9835	0.3442	−4.0213	0.3144
$\beta_{21}(-3)$	−3.0036	0.1409	−3.0039	0.1697	−3.0117	0.1667
$\beta_{02}(3)$	3.0017	0.0607	2.9863	0.0878	2.9925	0.0794
$\beta_{12}(7)$	6.9975	0.0977	7.0080	0.1199	7.0008	0.1251
$\beta_{22}(2)$	2.0013	0.0470	2.0037	0.0591	2.0016	0.0560
$\sigma_1^2(2)$	1.9416	0.4546	1.9680	0.5810	1.9397	0.5642
$\sigma_2^2(1)$	0.9820	0.1431	0.9517	0.1717	0.9589	0.1680
$\lambda_1(2)$	2.1293	1.0379	2.1125	0.8213	2.0707	0.9563
$\lambda_2(4)$	4.1458	1.2514	3.8421	1.0230	3.7720	1.0586
$\nu(3)$	–	–	3.0142	0.4777	3.3427	1.2521
$p_1(0.3)$	0.2998	0.0207	0.3002	0.0205	0.3008	0.0211

True values of parameters are in parentheses

Table 6.2 Scenario 2: mean and standard deviations (SD) for EM estimates based on 500 samples from the SMSN-MRM

	SN ($\Gamma_1 = \Gamma_2$)		ST ($\Gamma_1 = \Gamma_2$)		SSL($\Gamma_1 = \Gamma_2$)	
Parameter	Mean	SD	Mean	SD	Mean	SD
$\beta_{01}(-1)$	−1.0091	0.1778	−1.0370	0.2346	−0.9973	0.2055
$\beta_{11}(-4)$	−3.9832	0.2958	−4.0005	0.3386	−4.0235	0.3355
$\beta_{21}(-3)$	−3.0051	0.1431	−3.0016	0.1707	−3.0057	0.1814
$\beta_{02}(3)$	2.9882	0.1065	2.9836	0.1540	2.9915	0.1306
$\beta_{12}(7)$	7.0193	0.1812	7.0125	0.2246	7.0082	0.2165
$\beta_{22}(2)$	2.0093	0.0997	1.9978	0.1127	1.996	0.1100
$\sigma_1^2(2)$	1.8959	0.4086	1.8088	0.5414	1.8030	0.5421
$\sigma_2^2(2)$	1.9306	0.2674	1.9085	0.3992	1.8528	0.4462
$\lambda_1(2)$	1.8414	0.5898	1.8268	0.5598	1.6561	0.6370
$\lambda_2(2)$	1.8951	0.4690	1.9110	0.4608	1.7116	0.5301
$\nu(3)$	–	–	3.0070	0.5075	3.5332	1.8907
$p_1(0.3)$	0.2997	0.0216	0.2981	0.0219	0.3013	0.0204

True values of parameters are in parentheses

investigate the ability of the SMSN-MRM to cluster observations, that is, to allocate them into groups of observations that are similar in some sense. We know that each data point belongs to one of G heterogeneous populations, but we do not know how to discriminate between them. Modeling by mixture models allows clustering of the data in terms of the estimated (posterior) probability that a single point belongs to a given group.

A lot of work in model-based clustering has been done using finite mixtures of normal distributions. As the posterior probabilities $\widehat{z}_{ij}$, defined in (6.10), can be highly influenced by atypical observations, have been efforts to develop robust alternatives, like mixtures of t-Student distributions (see McLachlan and Peel 1998 and the references herein). Our idea is to extend the flexibility of these models, by including possible skewness of the related components; see the work of Liu and Lin (2014) based on the SN-MRM.

We generated 500 samples under the following scenarios: (a) scenario 1 (Fig. 6.1): a mixture of two skew-Birnbaum-Saunders regression models (see Santana et al. 2011; Vilca et al. 2011); and (b) scenario 2 (Fig. 6.2): a mixture of two skew-normal generalized hyperbolic models (see Vilca et al. 2014). The parameter values were chosen to present a considerable proportion of outliers and the skewness pattern. It can be seen from Figs. 6.1 and 6.2 that the groups are poorly separated. Furthermore, note that although we have a two-component mixture, the histogram need not be bimodal.

For each sample of size $n = 500$, we proceed with clustering ignoring the known true classification. Following the method proposed by Liu and Lin (2014), to assess the quality of the classification function of each mixture model, an index measure was used in the current study, called correct classification rate (CCR), which is based on the posterior probability assigned to each subject. The SMSN-MRM were fitted

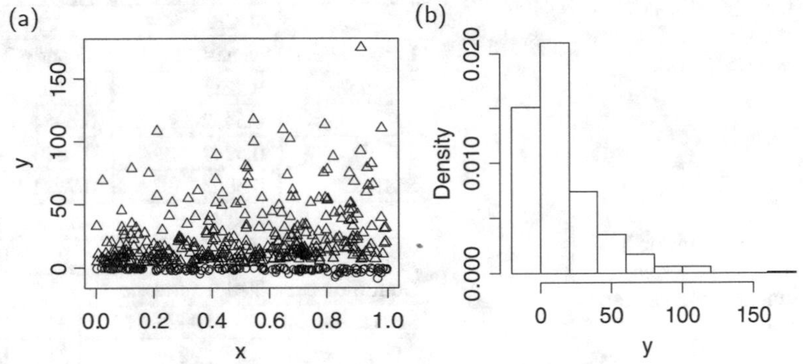

Fig. 6.1 Experiment 2. (**a**) The scatter plot and (**b**) histogram for one of the simulated samples—scenario 1

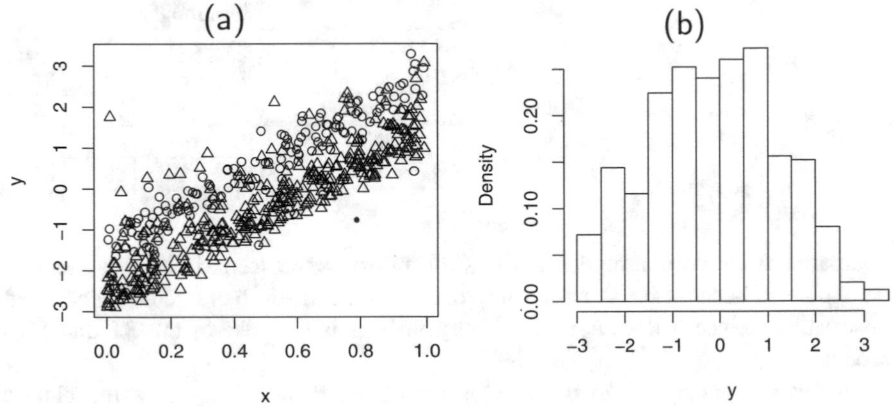

Fig. 6.2 Experiment 2. (**a**) The scatter plot and (**b**) histogram for one of the simulated samples—scenario 2

using the algorithm described in Sect. 6.2.1 in order to obtain the estimate of the posterior probability that an observation y_i belongs to the jth component of the mixture, i.e. $\widehat{z}_{ij}$. For sample l, $l = 1, \ldots, 500$, we compute the number of correct allocations (CCRs) divided by the sample size n, that is, $ACCR = \frac{1}{500}\sum_{l=1}^{500} CCR_l$. Table 6.3 shows the mean value of the correct allocation rates, where larger values indicate better classification results.

Obviously, one expects the best classification rate when modeling with true components (scenarios 1 and 2), but it is interesting to verify what happens when we use SMSN components. Comparing with the results for the normal model, we see that modeling using the ST or SSL distribution represents an improvement in the outright clustering and has a better performance, showing their robustness to discrepant observations. Under scenario 1, the SN model showed better performance

Table 6.3 Experiment 2. Mean of right allocation rates for fitted SMSN-MRM

	ACCR	
Fitted model	Scenario 1	Scenario 2
Normal	0.5211	0.7391
SN	0.5432	0.6964
ST	0.5747	0.7674
SSL	0.5603	0.7634

Table 6.4 Experiment 2. Percentages of preferred models under five conditions examined

	AIC	BIC	EDC	ICL
Condition examined	*Scenario 1*			
SN vs. normal	94	77	87	96
ST vs. normal	92	74	84	99
SSL vs. normal	73	43	57	99
ST vs. SN	62	62	62	99
SSL vs. SN	17	17	17	99
	Scenario 2			
SN vs. normal	79	21	41	51
ST vs. normal	93	65	77	81
SSL vs. normal	92	59	73	78
ST vs. SN	91	91	91	88
SSL vs. SN	88	88	88	85

compared to the normal model, but this did not occur in scenario 2. This fact can be explained because the skew-normal distribution can still be affected by atypical observations since it does not have heavy tails as is the case of the ST and SSL models.

For each sample of size $n = 500$, we compare the ability of some classic model selection criteria to select the appropriate model between the SMSN-MRM. Table 6.4 presents the percentages of models selected according to the four aforementioned criteria under five conditions, say, SN vs. Normal; ST vs. Normal; SSL vs. Normal; ST vs. SN; SSL vs. SN.

Under scenario 1 (data generated from a mixture of two skew-Birnbaum-Saunders regression models), comparing the asymmetric models SN, ST, and SSL with the normal (symmetrical) model, note that all criteria favor the asymmetric models (except the BIC when examining SSL vs. Normal). Moreover, note that the ICL criterion has the highest percentage since in this scenario the asymmetric models also performed better in classification (see Table 6.3). Comparing the asymmetric models with heavy tails (ST and SSL) to the SN model, the ST model was selected by all criteria.

Under scenario 2 (a mixture of two skew-normal generalized hyperbolic models), comparing the asymmetric models SN, ST, and SSL with normal symmetrical model, note that all criteria favor the asymmetric models (excluding BIC and EDC criteria in condition when examining SN vs. Normal). Note that when comparing SN vs. Normal, the ICL favors the SN model but the number of right allocations

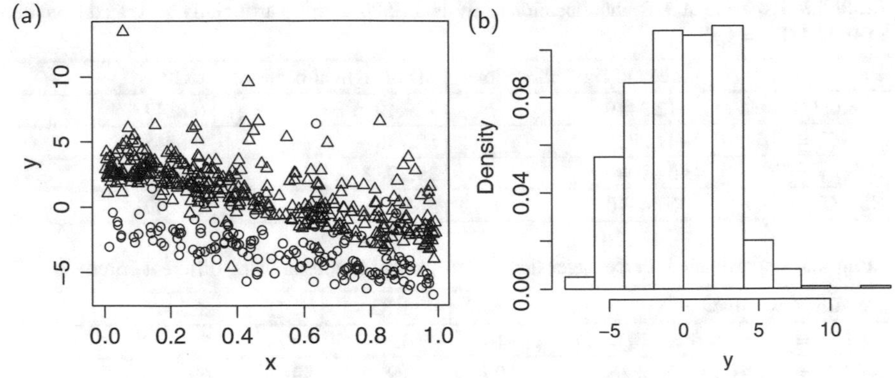

Fig. 6.3 Experiment 3. (**a**) The scatter plot and (**b**) histogram for one of the simulated samples

is greater for the normal model (see Table 6.3). Furthermore, for all criteria, the asymmetric models with heavy tails (ST and SSL) fitted the data better than the SN model.

6.3.3 Experiment 3: Classification

In this section, first we investigate the ability of the SMSN-MRM to cluster observations and then we compare the ability of some classic procedures to choose between the underlying SMSN-MRM. We fixed the number of components ($G = 2$), sample size ($n = 500$), and parameter values ($\boldsymbol{\beta}_1 = (-1, -4)^\top, \boldsymbol{\beta}_2 = (4, -6)^\top, \sigma_1^2 = \sigma_2^2 = 2, \lambda_1 = \lambda_2 = 2$, i.e, $\Gamma_1 = \Gamma_2$, and $p_1 = 0.3$), which is a restriction suggested by Basso et al. (2010) and Yao et al. (2014). Then, without loss of generality, we artificially generated 500 samples from a mixture regression of skew-t ($\nu = 3$) and, for each sample, we fitted the normal, SN, ST, and the SSL models with homogeneous nature of the covariance structure. Figure 6.3 shows a scatter plot and a histogram for one of these simulated samples.

From the clustering standpoint, in order to give stronger evidence of the superiority of the method using the SMSN-MRM family, the right number of allocations was computed for each sample. The mean and standard deviation (SD) of right allocations of these samples are shown in Table 6.5. It can be seen that the means are greater and the standard deviations are smaller for the skewed/heavy-tailed SMSN-MRM, in particular to the true model, i.e., ST model ($\Gamma_1 = \Gamma_2$). In addition, we present the mean value of the correct allocation rates ($ACCR$). Compared with the results for the normal model, modeling using the SN, ST, or SSL distribution represents a substantial improvement in the outright clustering. Also, the ST model (true model) outperforms performance when compared with the SN and the SSL models, as expected.

Table 6.5 Experiment 3. Right allocation analysis for 500 samples artificially generated from the ST model ($\Gamma_1 = \Gamma_2$)

Fitted model	Mean of right allocations	SD of right allocations	CCR
Normal ($\Gamma_1 = \Gamma_2$)	412.3440	109.4916	0.8247
SN ($\Gamma_1 = \Gamma_2$)	442.2720	58.7987	0.8845
ST ($\Gamma_1 = \Gamma_2$)	464.9040	39.3982	0.9298
SSL ($\Gamma_1 = \Gamma_2$)	457.4340	53.9565	0.9149

Table 6.6 Experiment 3. Percentages that the true model is chosen using different criteria

Condition examined	AIC	BIC	EDC	ICL
ST ($\Gamma_1 = \Gamma_2$) vs normal ($\Gamma_1 = \Gamma_2$)	100	100	100	5
ST ($\Gamma_1 = \Gamma_2$) vs SN ($\Gamma_1 = \Gamma_2$)	99	99	99	60
ST ($\Gamma_1 = \Gamma_2$) vs SSL ($\Gamma_1 = \Gamma_2$)	99	99	99	86

For each fitted model, we computed the AIC, BIC, EDC, and the ICL criterion. Table 6.6 shows the rates (percentages) at which the true model is chosen for each criterion. Note that all the criteria have satisfactory behavior, in that, they favor the true model, that is, the ST model with two components, except ICL which still performs poorly. Figure 6.4 shows the AIC values for each sample and model.

This simulation study shows similar results to those reported in Basso et al. (2010), in the context of mixture modeling based on scale mixtures of skew-normal distributions. We believe that this topic about model selection deserves a more detailed and extensive investigation, which is one of our purposes in order to extend the present paper including a study about the choice of the (possibly) unknown number of components, for example, and also treating the multivariate case. An overview of selection criteria can be found in Depraetere and Vandebroek (2014), in the context of mixture regression models based on the assumption of normality.

In addition, a real data set is analyzed, illustrating the usefulness of the proposed method. Thus, in the following application, we use those criteria as a rough guide for model choice.

6.4 Real Dataset

We illustrate our proposed methods with a dataset obtained from Cohen (1984), representing the perception of musical tones by musicians. In this perception experiment a pure fundamental tone with electronically generated overtones added was played to a trained musician. The subjects were asked to tune an adjustable tone to one octave above the fundamental tone and their perceived tone was recorded versus the actual tone. The experiment recorded 150 trials from the same musician. The overtones were determined by a stretching ratio, which is the ratio between adjusted tone and the fundamental tone. Two separate trends clearly emerge, see

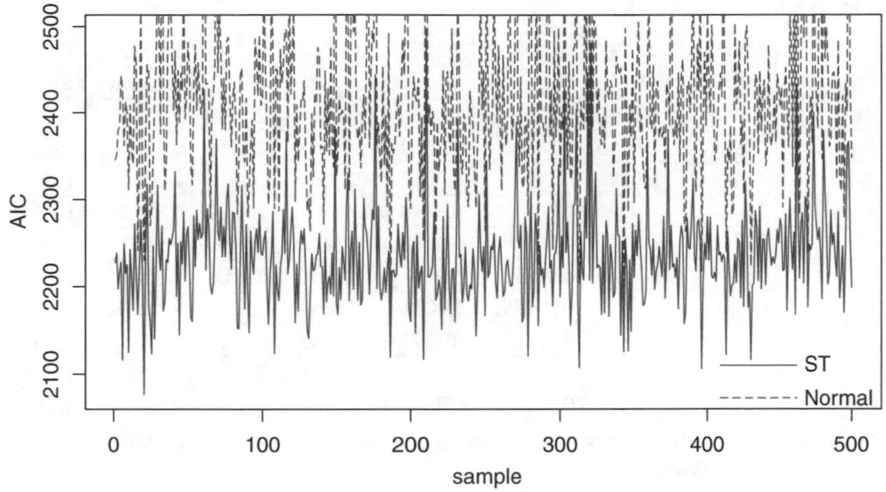

Fig. 6.4 Experiment 3. AIC values for 500 samples. Red line: ST model ($\Gamma_1 = \Gamma_2$) and blue line: Normal model ($\Gamma_1 = \Gamma_2$)

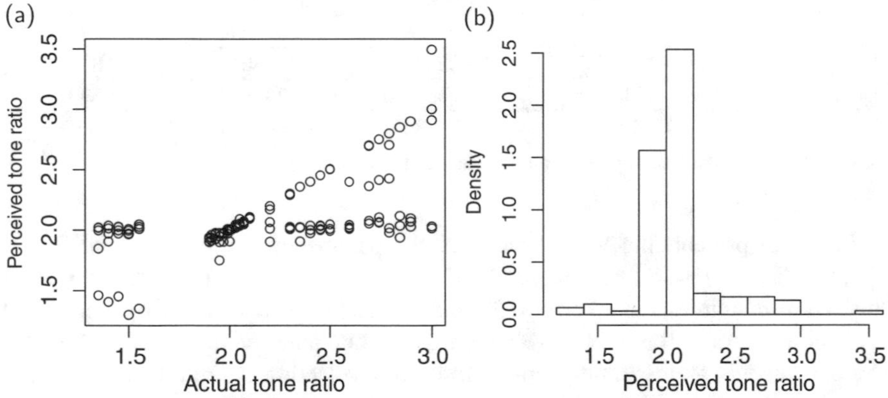

Fig. 6.5 (**a**) The scatter plot and (**b**) histogram of the tone perception data

Fig. 6.5a, which relate to two hypotheses explored in Cohen (1984), called the interval memory hypothesis and the partial matching hypothesis. Many articles have analyzed this dataset using a mixture of linear regressions framework; see DeVeaux (1989), Viele and Tong (2002), and Hunter and Young (2012). These data were analyzed recently by Yao et al. (2014), leading them to propose a robust mixture regression using the t-distribution. Now we revisit this dataset with the aim of expanding the inferential results to the SMSN family. Specifically, we focus on the SN, ST, and the SSL distributions. To verify the existence of skewness in the data, Fig. 6.5b presents a histogram of the data, showing an apparent non-normal pattern.

Table 6.7 Tone perception data

	Normal ($\Gamma_1 = \Gamma_2$)		SN ($\Gamma_1 = \Gamma_2$)		ST ($\Gamma_1 = \Gamma_2$)		SSL ($\Gamma_1 = \Gamma_2$)	
Parameter	Estimates	SE	Estimates	SE	Estimates	SE	Estimates	SE
β_{01}	1.8901	0.0399	1.9147	0.0236	1.9103	0.5490	1.9243	0.7695
β_{11}	0.0572	0.0175	0.0433	0.0109	0.0354	0.2768	0.0383	0.0163
β_{02}	−0.0442	0.0648	0.1594	0.0642	0.0019	0.5492	0.2061	0.0855
β_{12}	1.0111	0.0290	0.9044	0.0298	0.9978	0.2770	0.8859	0.3541
σ_1^2	0.0070	0.0008	0.0023	0.0003	0.0029	0.0008	0.0022	0.0010
σ_2^2	0.0070	0.0008	0.0793	0.0114	0.0001	0.0008	0.0541	0.0215
λ_1	–	–	−0.0128	0.0036	−8.0653	2.3243	−1.6120	0.6762
λ_2	–	–	5.7922	0.6347	−0.7363	2.1018	9.2738	3.8378
ν	–	–	–	–	2.0000	0.0439	2.0000	0.8752
$\mathbf{p}_1$	0.6765	0.0472	0.7310	0.0441	0.5496	0.0385	0.7251	0.2813

ML estimation results for fitting several mixture models. SE are the estimated standard errors based on the bootstrap procedure

Table 6.8 Tone perception data

Information criteria	Normal ($\Gamma_1 = \Gamma_2$)	SN ($\Gamma_1 = \Gamma_2$)	ST ($\Gamma_1 = \Gamma_2$)	SSL ($\Gamma_1 = \Gamma_2$)
Log-likelihood	106.2549	134.0726	**201.2834**	135.5021
AIC	−198.5097	−250.1451	**−382.5667**	−251.0041
BIC	−174.4247	−220.0387	**−352.4604**	−220.8977
EDC	−194.9138	−245.6502	**−378.0718**	−246.5092
ICL	4274.6590	6831.2690	**1299.2110**	1318.8930

Some information criteria. The bold values indicates the best fitted model

Table 6.7 presents the ML estimates of the parameters from the normal ($\Gamma_1 = \Gamma_2$), SN ($\Gamma_1 = \Gamma_2$), ST ($\Gamma_1 = \Gamma_2$), and the SSL ($\Gamma_1 = \Gamma_2$) models, along with their corresponding standard errors (SE) calculated via the bootstrap procedure (100 replications). As in Basso et al. (2010), we also compare the normal, SN, ST, and the SSL models by inspecting some information selection criteria. Comparing the models by looking at the values of the information criteria presented in Table 6.8, we observe that the SN, ST, and the SSL models outperform the normal model, indicating that asymmetric distributions with heavier tails provide a better fit than the normal and the SN distributions. In addition, it appears that the ST model presents a better fit than all other models.

For this dataset we also adjusted the normal, SN, ST, and the SSL models without considering the homogeneous nature of the variance parameter, but the ST ($\Gamma_1 = \Gamma_2$) model showed the best fit compared to other models. Thus, for brevity we present only the results for the models with homogeneous nature of the scale parameter.

From the clustering point of view, in order to give evidence of the superiority of the method using the SMSN-MRM family, we carried out a bootstrap experiment with 100 replications. For each replication, the right number of allocations was computed. The mean and standard deviation (SD) of these bootstrap replications

Table 6.9 Tone perception data

Fitted model	Mean of RA	SD of RA	95% IC for RA
Normal	130.9500	3.4275	[124.0095;137.8005]
SN	136.7900	6.8199	[123.1502;150.4298]
ST	141.4000	2.7303	[135.9394;146.8606]
SSL	138.6264	3.3071	[132.0122;145.2406]

Right allocation (RA) analysis through bootstrap procedure for the dataset

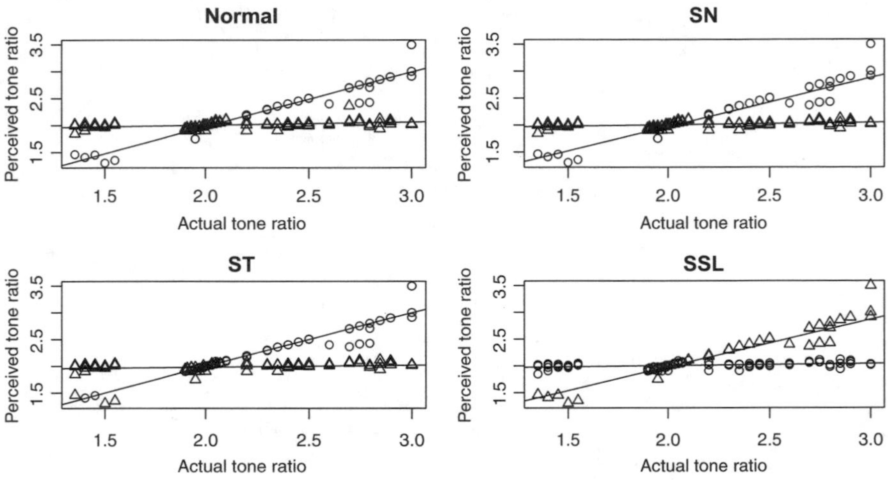

Fig. 6.6 Tone perception data. The scatter plots of the dataset with the fitted models

are shown in Table 6.9. Also, we present the associated 95% normal asymptotic confidence intervals (IC). It can be seen that the means are greater and the standard deviations are smaller for the heavy-tailed SMSN-MRM. Figure 6.6 shows the scatter plots of the data set with the fitted models.

References

Aitkin, M., & Wilson, G. T. (1980). Mixture models, outliers, and the EM algorithm. *Technometrics, 22*, 325–331. 19

Akaike, H. (1974). A new look at the statistical model identification. *IEEE Transactions on Automatic Control, 19*, 716–723. 3, 49

Andrews, D. F., & Mallows, C. L. (1974). Scale mixtures of normal distributions. *Journal of the Royal Statistical Society, Series B, 36*, 99–102. 15, 15, 17, 78

Arellano-Valle, R. B., Bolfarine, H., & Lachos, V. H. (2005). Skew-normal linear mixed models. *Journal of Data Science, 3*, 415–438. 22

Arellano-Valle, R. B., Castro, L. M., Genton, M. G., & Gómez, H. W. (2008). Bayesian inference for shape mixtures of skewed distributions, with application to regression analysis. *Bayesian Analysis, 3*, 513–539. 78

Arellano-Valle, R. B., del Pino, G., & Martín, E. S. (2002). Definition and probabilistic properties of skew-distributions. *Statistics & Probability Letters, 58*, 111–121. 17

Arnold, B. C., Beaver, R. J., Groeneveld, R. A., & Meeker, W. Q. (1993). The nontruncated marginal of a truncated bivariate normal distribution. *Psychometrika, 58*, 471–488. 42

Azzalini, A. (1985). A class of distributions which includes the normal ones. *Scandinavian Journal of Statistics, 12*, 171–178. 16, 58, 78

Azzalini, A. (2005). The skew-normal distribution and related multivariate families. *Scandinavian Journal of Statistics, 32*, 159–188. 42

Azzalini, A., & Capitanio, A. (1999). Statistical applications of the multivariate skew-normal distribution. *Journal of the Royal Statistical Society, 61*, 579–602. 24, 25

Azzalini, A., & Capitanio, A. (2003). Distributions generated by perturbation of symmetry with emphasis on a multivariate skew t-distribution. *Journal of the Royal Statistical Society, Series B, 65*, 367–389. 17, 17, 26, 58, 78

Azzalini, A., & Dalla-Valle, A. (1996). The multivariate skew-normal distribution. *Biometrika, 83*, 715–726. 16, 16, 17, 17, 58

Bai, Z. D., Krishnaiah, P. R., & Zhao, L. C. (1989). On rates of convergence of efficient detection criteria in signal processing with white noise. *IEEE Transactions on Automatic Control, 35*, 380–388. 52, 52

Basford, K. E., Greenway, D. R., Mclachlan, G. J., & Peel, D. (1997). Standard errors of fitted component means of normal mixtures. *Computational Statistics, 12*, 1–17. 63, 67

Basso, R. M., Lachos, V. H., Cabral, C. R. B., & Ghosh, P. (2010). Robust mixture modeling based on scale mixtures of skew-normal distributions. *Computational Statistics and Data Analysis, 54*, 2926–2941. 37, 58, 58, 74, 78, 82, 83, 84, 89, 90, 92

V. H. Lachos Dávila et al., *Finite Mixture of Skewed Distributions*,
SpringerBriefs in Statistics, https://doi.org/10.1007/978-3-319-98029-4

Biernacki, C., Celeux, G., & Govaert, G. (2000). Assessing a mixture model for clustering with the integrated completed likelihood. *IEEE Transactions on Pattern Analysis and Machine Intelligence, 22*, 719–725. 52, 54, 74

Biernacki, C., & Govaert, G. C. G. (2003). Choosing starting values for the EM algorithm for getting the highest likelihood in multivariate Gaussian mixture models. *Computational Statistics & Data Analysis, 41*, 561–575. 37

Böhning, D. (2000). *Computer-assisted analysis of mixtures and applications. Meta-analysis, disease mapping and others*. Boca Raton: Chapman&Hall/CRC. 1

Böhning, D., Hennig, C., McLachlan, G. J., & McNicholas, P. D. (2014). Editorial: The 2nd special issue on advances in mixture models. *Computational Statistics & Data Analysis, 71*, 1–2. 1, 7

Böhning, D., & Seidel, W. (2003). Editorial: Recent developments in mixture models. *Computational Statistics & Data Analysis, 41*, 349–357. Recent Developments in Mixture Model. 7

Böhning, D., Seidel, W., Alfó, M., Garel, B., Patilea, V., & Walther, G. (2007). Editorial: Advances in mixture models. *Computational Statistics & Data Analysis, 51*, 5205–5210. Recent Developments in Mixture Model. 7

Branco, M. D., & Dey, D. K. (2001). A general class of multivariate skew-elliptical distributions. *Journal of Multivariate Analysis, 79*, 99–113. vii, 15, 17, 58, 78

Cabral, C. R. B., Bolfarine, H., & Pereira, J. R. G. (2008). Bayesian density estimation using skew Student-t-normal mixtures. *Computational Statistics & Data Analysis, 52*, 5075–5090. 58

Cabral, C. R. B., Lachos, V. H., & Prates, M. O. (2012). Multivariate mixture modeling using skew-normal independent distributions. *Computational Statistics and Data Analysis, 56*, 126–142. 57, 58

Charlier, C. V. L., & Wicksell, S. D. (1924). On the dissection of frequency functions. *Arkiv för Matematik, Astronomi och Fysik, 18*, 1–64. 7

Cohen, E. (1984). Some effects of inharmonic partials on interval perception. *Music Perception, 1*, 323–349. 90, 91

Cosslett, S. R., & Lee, L.-F. (1985). Serial correlation in latent discrete variable models. *Journal of Econometrics, 27*, 79–97. 78

DasGupta, A. (2008). *Asymptotic theory of statistics and probability*. New York: Springer. 2

Dempster, A. P., Laird, N. M., & Rubin, D. B. (1977). Maximum likelihood from incomplete data via the EM algorithm. *Journal of the Royal Statistical Society, Series B, 39*, 1–38. 7, 8, 37, 57, 78, 80

Depraetere, N., & Vandebroek, M. (2014). Order selection in finite mixtures of linear regressions. *Statistical Papers, 55*, 871–911. 90

DeSarbo, W. S., & Cron, W. L. (1988). A maximum likelihood methodology for clusterwise linear regression. *Journal of Classification, 5*, 248–282. 78

DeSarbo, W. S., Wedel, M., Vriens, M., & Ramaswamy, V. (1992). Latent class metric conjoint analysis. *Marketing Letters, 3*, 273–288. 78

DeVeaux, R. D. (1989). Mixtures of linear regressions. *Computational Statistics and Data Analysis, 8*. 227–245. 91

Dias, J. G., & Wedel, M. (2004). An empirical comparison of EM, SEM and MCMC performance for problematic Gaussian mixture likelihoods. *Statistics and Computing, 14*, 323–332. 37, 41, 62

DiCiccio, T. J., & Monti, A. C. (2004). Inferential aspects of the skew exponential power distribution. *Journal of the American Statistical Association, 99*, 439–450. 49

Doetsch, G. (1928). Die elimination des dopplereffekts bei spektroskopischen feinstrukturen und exakte bestimmung der komponenten. *Zeitschrift für Physik, 49*, 705–730. 7

Doğru, F. Z., & Arslan, O. (2017). Robust mixture regression based on the skew t distribution. *Revista Colombiana de Estadística, 40*, 45–64. 78

Efron, B., & Tibshirani, R. (1986). Bootstrap methods for standard errors, confidence intervals, and other measures of statistical accuracy. *Statistical Science, 1*, 54–75. 46, 66

Frank, A., & Asuncion, A. (2010). *UCI machine learning repository*. 74

Frühwirth-Schnatter, S. (2006). *Finite mixture and Markov switching models*. New York: Springer. 1, 1, 60, 78

Gentle, J. E. (2007). *Matrix algebra: Theory, computations, and applications in statistics*. New York: Springer. 16

Genton, M. G., He, L., & Liu, X. (2001). Moments of skew-normal random vectors and their quadratic forms. *Statistics & Probability Letters, 51*(4), 319–325. 24

Greselin, F., & Ingrassia, S. (2010). Constrained monotone EM algorithms for mixtures of multivariate t distributions. *Statistics and Computing, 20*, 9–22. 76

Gruen, B. (2015). *Bayesmix: Bayesian Mixture Models with JAGS*. R package version 0.7-4. 1

Gupta, A. (2003). Multivariate skew t-distribution. *Statistics, 37*(4), 359–363. 17, 25, 26

Hamilton, J. D. (1989). A new approach to the economic analysis of nonstationary time series and the business cycle. *Econometrica: Journal of the Econometric Society, 57*, 357–384 78

Hartigan, J. A., & Wong, M. A. (1979). A k-means clustering algorithm. *Applied Statistics, 28*, 100–108. 42

Hasselblad, V. (1966). Estimation of parameters for a mixture of normal distributions. *Technometrics, 8*, 431–444. 7

Hasselblad, V. (1969). Estimation of finite mixtures of distributions from the exponential family. *Journal of the American Statistical Association, 64*, 1459–1471. 7

Hathaway, R. J. (1985). A constrained formulation of maximum-likelihood estimation for normal mixture models. *The Annals of Statistics, 13*, 795–800. 76

Holzmann, H., Munk, A., & Gneiting, T. (2006). Identifiability of finite mixtures of elliptical distributions. *Scandinavian Journal of Statistics, 33*, 753–763. 76

Hunter, D. R., & Young, D. S. (2012). Semiparametric mixtures of regressions. *Journal of Nonparametric Statistics, 24*(1), 19–38. 91

Ingrassia, S. (2004). A likelihood-based constrained algorithm for multivariate normal mixture models. *Statistical Methods and Applications, 13*, 151–166. 76

Ingrassia, S., & Rocci, R. (2007). Constrained monotone EM algorithms for finite mixture of multivariate Gaussians. *Computational Statistics & Data Analysis, 51*, 5339–5351. 76

Karlis, D., & Santourian, A. (2009). Model-based clustering with non-elliptically contoured distributions. *Statistics and Computing, 19*, 73–83. 63, 71, 72

Lachos, V. H., Bolfarine, H., Arellano-Valle, R. B., & Montenegro, L. C. (2007). Likelihood based inference for multivariate skew-normal regression models. *Communications in Statistics-Theory and Methods, 36*, 1769–1786. 31, 34

Lachos, V. H., Ghosh, P., & Arellano-Valle, R. B. (2010). Likelihood based inference for skew-normal independent linear mixed models. *Statistica Sinica, 20*, 303–322. vii, 20, 23, 44, 58, 78

Lange, K. L., Little, R., & Taylor, J. (1989). Robust statistical modeling using t distribution. *Journal of the American Statistical Association, 84*, 881–896. 18

Lange, K. L., & Sinsheimer, J. S. (1993). Normal/independent distributions and their applications in robust regression. *Journal of Computational and Graphical Statistics, 2*, 175–198. vii, 17, 17, 18, 20, 25, 32, 58

Lee, S., & McLachlan, G. J. (2014). Finite mixtures of multivariate skew t-distributions: some recent and new results. *Statistics and Computing, 24*(2), 181–202. 57

Lee, S. X., & McLachlan, G. J. (2013). On mixtures of skew normal and skew t-distributions. *Advances in Data Analysis and Classification, 7*(3), 241–266. 57

Lee, S. X., & McLachlan, G. J. (2016). Finite mixtures of canonical fundamental skew t-distributions. *Statistics and Computing, 26*(3), 573–589. 57

Lehmann, E. L. (1999). *Elements of large-sample theory*. New York: Springer. 10

Lin, T. I. (2009). Maximum likelihood estimation for multivariate skew normal mixture models. *Journal of Multivariate Analysis, 100*, 257–265. 31, 57, 58, 63

Lin, T. I. (2010). Robust mixture modeling using multivariate skew t distributions. *Statistics and Computing, 20*, 343–356. 31, 57, 58, 63, 63

Lin, T. I., Lee, J. C., & Hsieh, W. J. (2007a). Robust mixture modelling using the skew t distribution. *Statistics and Computing, 17*, 81–92. 37, 37, 41, 54, 54, 54, 58

Lin, T. I., Lee, J. C., & Ni, H. F. (2004). Bayesian analysis of mixture modelling using the multivariate t distribution. *Statistics and Computing, 14*, 119–130. 57

Lin, T. I., Lee, J. C., & Yen, S. Y. (2007b). Finite mixture modelling using the skew normal distribution. *Statistica Sinica, 17*, 909–927. 37, 37, 41, 42, 58

Lin, T.-I., Wang, W.-L., McLachlan, G. J., & Lee, S. X. (2018). Robust mixtures of factor analysis models using the restricted multivariate skew-t distribution. *Statistical Modelling, 28*, 50–72. 57

Lindsay, B. G. (1995). *Mixture models: Theory geometry and applications*, volume 51. NSF-CBMS Regional Conference Series in Probability and Statistics, Institute of Mathematical Statistics, Hayward. 1

Little, R. J. (1988). Robust estimation of the mean and covariance matrix from data with missing values. *Applied Statistics, 37*, 23–38. 18

Liu, M., Hancock, G. R., & Harring, J. R. (2011). Using finite mixture modeling to deal with systematic measurement error: A case study. *Journal of Modern Applied Statistical Methods, 10*, 22. 78

Liu, M., & Lin, T.-I. (2014). A skew-normal mixture regression model. *Educational and Psychological Measurement, 74*, 139–162. 77, 78, 78, 79, 86, 86

Liu, C., & Rubin, D. B. (1994). The ECME algorithm: A simple extension of EM and ECM with faster monotone convergence. *Biometrika, 80*, 267–278. 37, 78

Mardia, K. V. (1970). Measures of multivariate skewness and kurtosis with applications. *Biometrika, 657*, 519–530. 24

McLachlan, G., Bean, R., & Jones, L. B. T. (2007). Extension of the mixture of factor analyzers model to incorporate the multivariate t-distribution. *Computational Statistics & Data Analysis, 51*, 5327–5338. 76

McLachlan, G. J., & Basford, K. E. (1988). *Mixture models: Inference and applications to clustering*. New York: Marcel Dekker. 13

McLachlan, G. J., & Krishnan, T. (2008). *The EM algorithm and extensions*, 2nd ed. New York: Wiley. 8, 37, 57, 82

McLachlan, G. J., & Peel, D. (1998). Robust cluster analysis via mixtures of multivariate t-distributions. *Lecture Notes in Computer Science, 1451*, 658–666. 46, 86

McLachlan, G. J., & Peel, D. (2000). *Finite mixture models*. New York: Wiley. 1, 7, 11, 37, 54, 57, 59, 71, 73, 78, 80, 85

Meng, X., & Rubin, D. B. (1993). Maximum likelihood estimation via the ECM algorithm: A general framework. *Biometrika, 81*, 633–648. 37, 78

Mengersen, K., Robert, C. P., & Titterington, D. M. (2011). *Mixtures: Estimation and applications*. New York: Wiley. 1

Nityasuddhi, D., & Böhning, D. (2003). Asymptotic properties of the EM algorithm estimate for normal mixture models with component specific variances. *Computational Statistics & Data Analysis, 41*, 591–601. 37, 49, 60

Pearson, K. (1894). Contribution to the mathematical theory of evolution. *Philosophical Transactions A, 185*, 71–110. 7

Peel, D., & McLachlan, G. J. (2000). Robust mixture modelling using the t distribution. *Statistics and Computing, 10*, 339–348. 37

Prates, M. O., Cabral, C. R. B., & Lachos, V. H. (2013). mixsmsn: Fitting finite mixture of scale mixture of skew-normal distributions. *Journal of Statistical Software, 54*, 1–20. 3, 37, 57, 58, 58, 66, 84

Punathumparambath, B. (2012). The multivariate skew-slash t and skew-slash Cauchy distributions. *Model Assisted Statistics and Applications, 7*, 33–40. 17

Pyne, S., Hu, X., Wang, K., Rossin, E., Lin, T., Baecher-Allan, L. M. M. C., McLachlan, G. J. P., Tamayo, D. A. H., De Jager, P. L., & Mesirov, J. P. (2009). Automated high-dimensional flow cytometric data analysis. *Proceedings of the National Academy of Sciences USA, 106*, 8519–8524. 58

Quandt, R. E. (1972). A new approach to estimating switching regressions. *Journal of the American Statistical Association, 67*, 306–310. 78

Quandt, R. E., & Ramsey, J. B. (1978). Estimating mixtures of normal distributions and switching regressions. *Journal of the American Statistical Association, 73*, 730–738. 78

Rao, C. R. (1948). The utilization of multiple measurements in problems of biological classification. *Journal of the Royal Statistical Society. Series B (Methodological), 10*, 159–203. 7

Rogers, W. H., & Tukey, J. W. (1972). Understanding some long-tailed symmetrical distributions. *Statistica Neerlandica, 26*, 211–226. 18

Sahu, S. K., Dey, D. K., & Branco, M. D. (2003). A new class of multivariate skew distributions with applications to Bayesian regression models. *The Canadian Journal of Statistics, 31*, 129–150. 58

Santana, L., Vilca, F., & Leiva, V. (2011). Influence analysis in skew-Birnbaum-Saunders regression models and applications. *Journal of Applied Statistics, 38*, 1633–1649. 86

Schwarz, G. (1978). Estimating the dimension of a model. *Annals of Statistics, 6*, 461–464. 3, 49

Sfikas, G., Nikou, C., & Galatsanos, N. (2007). Robust image segmentation with mixtures of Student's t-distributions. *IEEE International Conference on Image Processing, 1*. ICIP 2007. 57

Shoham, S. (2002). Robust clustering by deterministic agglomeration EM of mixtures of multivariate t-distributions. *Pattern Recognition, 35*, 1127–1142. 57

Shoham, S., Fellows, M. R., & Normann, R. A. (2003). Robust automatic spike sorting using mixtures of multivariate t-distributions. *Journal of Neuroscience Methods, 127*, 111–122. 57

Späth, H. (1979). Algorithm 39 clusterwise linear regression. *Computing, 22*, 367–373. 78

Strömgren, B. (1934). Tables and diagrams for dissecting a frequency curve into components by the half-invariant method. *Scandinavian Actuarial Journal, 17*, 7–54. 7

Titterington, D. M., Smith, A. F. M., & Makov, U. E. (1985). *Statistical analysis of finite mixture distributions*. New York: Wiley. 1, 76

Turner, T. R. (2000). Estimating the propagation rate of a viral infection of potato plants via mixtures of regressions. *Journal of the Royal Statistical Society: Series C (Applied Statistics), 49*, 371–384. 78

Viele, K., & Tong, B. (2002). Modeling with mixtures of linear regressions. *Statistics and Computing, 12*, 315–330. 91

Vilca, F., Santana, L., Leiva, V., & Balakrishnan, N. (2011). Estimation of extreme percentiles in Birnbaum-Saunders distributions. *Computational Statistics and Data Analysis, 55*, 1665–1678. 86

Vilca, F., Balakrishnan, N., & Zeller, C. B. (2014). Multivariate skew-normal generalized hyperbolic distribution and its properties. *Journal of Multivariate Analysis, 128*, 73–85. 86

Wang, H. X., Zhang, Q. B., Luo, B., & Wei, S. (2004). Robust mixture modelling using multivariate t-distribution with missing information. *Pattern Recognition Letters, 25*, 701–710. 25, 57

Wang, J., & Genton, M. G. (2006). The multivariate skew-slash distribution. *Journal of Statistical Planning and Inference, 136*, 209–220. 17, 17, 27, 78

Wei, G. C. G., & Tanner, M. A. (1990). A Monte Carlo implementation of the EM algorithm and the poor man's data augmentation algorithms. *Journal of the American Statistical Association, 85*, 699–704. 82

Weldon, W. F. R. (1893). On certain correlated variations in *carcinus maenas*. *Proceedings of the Royal Society of London, 54*, 318–329. 7

Wolfe, J. H. (1965). A computer program for the maximum-likelihood analysis of types. Defense documentation center AD 620 026, U. S. Naval Personnel Research Activity. Technical Bulletin 65-15. 7

Wolfe, J. H. (1967). NORMIX: Computational methods for estimating the parameters of multivariate normal mixtures of distributions. Defense documentation center AD 656 588, U. S. Naval Personnel Research Activity. Research Memorandum SRM 68-2. 7

Yakowitz, S. J., & Spragins, J. D. (1968). On the identifiability of finite mixtures. *The Annals of Mathematical Statistics, 39*, 209–214. 76

Yao, W., Wei, Y., & Yu, C. (2014). Robust mixture regression using the t-distribution. *Computational Statistics and Data Analysis, 71*, 116–127. 77, 78, 78, 79, 83, 89, 91

Yu, C., Zhang, Q., & Guo, L. (2006). Robust clustering algorithms based on finite mixtures of multivariate t distribution. *Lecture Notes in Computer Science, 4221*, 606–609. 57

Zeller, C. B., Cabral, C. R. B., & Lachos, V. H. (2016). Robust mixture regression modeling based on scale mixtures of skew-normal distributions. *TEST, 25*, 375–396. 77

Zeller, C. B., Lachos, V. H., & Vilca-Labra, F. E. (2011). Local influence analysis for regression models with scale mixtures of skew-normal distributions. *Journal of Applied Statistics, 38*, 348–363. 82, 82

Index

V. H. Lachos Dávila et al., *Finite Mixture of Skewed Distributions*,
SpringerBriefs in Statistics, https://doi.org/10.1007/978-3-319-98029-4